DEADLY DISEASES AND EPIDEMICS

ENCEPHALITIS

DEADLY DISEASES AND EPIDEMICS

Anthrax

Botulism

Campylobacteriosis

Cholera

Ebola

Encephalitis

Escherichia coli Infections

Gonorrhea

Hepatitis

Herpes

HIV/AIDS

Human Papillomavirus and Warts

Influenza

Leprosy

Lyme Disease

Mad Cow Disease (Bovine Spongiform Encephalopathy)

Malaria

Meningitis

Mononucleosis

Pelvic Inflammatory Disease

Plague

Polio

Salmonella

SARS

Smallpox

Streptococcus (Group A)

Staphylococcus aureus Infections

Syphilis

Toxic Shock Syndrome

Tuberculosis

Typhoid Fever

West Nile Virus

DEADLY DISEASES AND EPIDEMICS

ENCEPHALITIS

Ona Bloom
and
Jennifer R. Morgan

FOUNDING EDITOR
The Late **I. Edward Alcamo**
Distinguished Teaching Professor of Microbiology,
SUNY Farmingdale

FOREWORD BY
David Heymann
World Health Organization

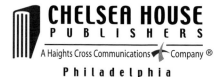

CHELSEA HOUSE
P U B L I S H E R S
A Haights Cross Communications Company ®
Philadelphia

CHELSEA HOUSE PUBLISHERS

VP, NEW PRODUCT DEVELOPMENT Sally Cheney
DIRECTOR OF PRODUCTION Kim Shinners
CREATIVE MANAGER Takeshi Takahashi
MANUFACTURING MANAGER Diann Grasse

Staff for Encephalitis

EXECUTIVE EDITOR Tara Koellhoffer
ASSOCIATE EDITOR Beth Reger
EDITORIAL ASSISTANT Kuorkor Dzani
PRODUCTION EDITOR Noelle Nardone
PHOTO EDITOR Sarah Bloom
SERIES DESIGNER Terry Mallon
COVER DESIGNER Keith Trego
LAYOUT 21st Century Publishing and Communications, Inc.

http://www.chelseahouse.com

First Printing

1 3 5 7 9 8 6 4 2

Library of Congress Cataloging-in-Publication Data

Bloom, Ona.
    Encephalitis /Ona Bloom and Jennifer Morgan.
       p. cm.—(Deadly diseases and epidemics)
    Includes bibliographical references and index.
    ISBN 0-7910-8503-1
    1. Encephalitis. I. Morgan, Jennifer, 1955- II. Title. III. Series.
RC390.B56 2005
616.8'32—dc22

                                                        2005005518

Table of Contents

Foreword

In the 1960s, many of the infectious diseases that had terrorized generations were tamed. After a century of advances, the leading killers of Americans both young and old were being prevented with new vaccines or cured with new medicines. The risk of death from pneumonia, tuberculosis (TB), meningitis, influenza, whooping cough, and diphtheria declined dramatically. New vaccines lifted the fear that summer would bring polio, and a global campaign was on the verge of eradicating smallpox worldwide. New pesticides like DDT cleared mosquitoes from homes and fields, thus reducing the incidence of malaria, which was present in the southern United States and which remains a leading killer of children worldwide. New technologies produced safe drinking water and removed the risk of cholera and other water-borne diseases. Science seemed unstoppable. Disease seemed destined to all but disappear.

But the euphoria of the 1960s has evaporated.

The microbes fought back. Those causing diseases like TB and malaria evolved resistance to cheap and effective drugs. The mosquito developed the ability to defuse pesticides. New diseases emerged, including AIDS, Legionnaires, and Lyme disease. And diseases which had not been seen in decades re-emerged, as the hantavirus did in the Navajo Nation in 1993. Technology itself actually created new health risks. The global transportation network, for example, meant that diseases like West Nile virus could spread beyond isolated regions and quickly become global threats. Even modern public health protections sometimes failed, as they did in 1993 in Milwaukee, Wisconsin, resulting in 400,000 cases of the digestive system illness cryptosporidiosis. And, more recently, the threat from smallpox, a disease believed to be completely eradicated, has returned along with other potential bioterrorism weapons such as anthrax.

The lesson is that the fight against infectious diseases will never end.

In our constant struggle against disease, we as individuals have a weapon that does not require vaccines or drugs, and that is the warehouse of knowledge. We learn from the history of science that "modern" beliefs can be wrong. In this series of books, for example, you will learn that diseases like syphilis were once thought to be caused by eating potatoes. The invention of the microscope set science on the right path. There are more positive lessons from history. For example, smallpox was eliminated by vaccinating everyone who had come in contact with an infected person. This "ring" approach to smallpox control is still the preferred method for confronting an outbreak, should the disease be intentionally reintroduced.

At the same time, we are constantly adding new drugs, new vaccines, and new information to the warehouse. Recently, the entire human genome was decoded. So too was the genome of the parasite that causes malaria. Perhaps by looking at the microbe and the victim through the lens of genetics we will be able to discover new ways to fight malaria, which remains the leading killer of children in many countries.

Because of advances in our understanding of such diseases as AIDS, entire new classes of anti-retroviral drugs have been developed. But resistance to all these drugs has already been detected, so we know that AIDS drug development must continue.

Education, experimentation, and the discoveries that grow out of them are the best tools to protect health. Opening this book may put you on the path of discovery. I hope so, because new vaccines, new antibiotics, new technologies, and, most importantly, new scientists are needed now more than ever if we are to remain on the winning side of this struggle against microbes.

David Heymann
Executive Director
Communicable Diseases Section
World Health Organization
Geneva, Switzerland

1

An Introduction to Viral Encephalitis

In August 1999, the New York City Department of Health and Mental Hygiene issued a total of one press release for the entire month—it was on the topic of AIDS. By the end of September 1999, the department had issued 26 press releases, 23 of which discussed topics related to the sudden rise in local cases of **encephalitis**, a severe inflammation of the brain. You can read the first of these press releases and a follow-up issued later in the month in the special feature box on page 10. As it turns out, the 1999 investigation, which began with eight cases of encephalitis in New York City, kicked off an intense monitoring of the surrounding areas. Subsequently, these cases were identified as the first outbreak of West Nile virus in the Western Hemisphere.

It all started during the warm days of late August in New York. An infectious disease doctor at a hospital in Queens made a call to the New York City Department of Health to report that two of his patients had encephalitis accompanied by profound muscle weakness—a relatively rare diagnosis. Another six cases of encephalitis were quickly identified in nearby hospitals, bringing the total to eight. All of the patients had some combination of the classic symptoms of encephalitis, including fever, abnormal mental status, such as confusion, disorientation, irritability, and drowsiness; severe headaches; and muscle weakness. Some patients were so weak, in fact, that they had to be put on a ventilator to help them breathe.

Samples of the patients' blood, spinal cord fluid, and tissues were collected and tested for signs of infection and various possible sources of encephalitis, which is most often caused by a **pathogen** (an infectious organism) such as a **virus**. Indeed, the test results suggested that the cause of the encephalitis was a viral infection. Scientists determined that the virus was either the St. Louis encephalitis virus, which is carried by mosquitoes and birds, or one closely related to it. At the same time, an unusual number of birds were found dead throughout the region. Some of the birds had also suffered from encephalitis, which seemed to be more than a coincidence. The virus that was found in the birds was also related to the St. Louis encephalitis virus; it was the same virus that had infected the people in the area. The virus was eventually identified as West Nile virus.

By the end of September 1999, 59 patients had been hospitalized in the greater New York metropolitan area with a similar viral infection, and most of these patients had symptoms of encephalitis. In 2003 alone, throughout the United States, there were close to 3,000 cases of encephalitis or **meningitis** (a swelling of the membranes that surround the brain and spinal cord) and 200 deaths caused by West Nile virus. Although this increase in the number of encephalitis cases occurring in the United States was (and still is) cause for concern, it pales in comparison to the 30,000–50,000 cases of encephalitis that occur in Asia each year, most of which are caused by a virus in the same family as the West Nile virus, called the Japanese encephalitis virus. The rapid spread of West Nile virus across the United States in just a few years makes it likely that the number of cases of encephalitis will continue to increase across North America (Figure 1.1).

As mentioned above, encephalitis refers to an acute inflammation of the brain. The word *encephalitis* is derived from the Greek word *enkephalos*, which means "in the head." **Encephalomyelitis** refers to an inflammation of both the brain and spinal cord. There are many different causes of encephalitis, but the most common is an infection by a virus or, in some cases, another pathogen such as a **bacterium**. The different

(continued on page 13)

PRESS RELEASE

New York City Department of Health Office of Public Affairs

IMMEDIATE RELEASE: Friday, September 3, 1999

CITY HEALTH DEPARTMENT REPORTS THREE CASES OF ST. LOUIS ENCEPHALITIS (SLE) IN QUEENS

Other Possible Cases Being Investigated

The New York City Department of Health (DOH) today reported that the death of one elderly individual and the illness of two other elderly persons in Queens were confirmed to be associated with St. Louis encephalitis (SLE), a viral disease transmitted by mosquitoes. While very few mosquitoes carry the SLE virus, Health Commissioner Neal L. Cohen, M.D., advised New York City residents, particularly those in the Whitestone/Flushing/Auburndale areas of Queens, to take immediate precautions to minimize the possibility of additional infections. Although cases of SLE sometimes occur in the Southeast United States, these are the first known cases of SLE to be acquired in New York City.

"Most people recover from St. Louis Encephalitis, but in some cases—especially among the elderly and children—it can be a serious and even fatal disease," Mayor Rudolph W. Giuliani said. "I want to thank the U.S. Centers for Disease Control and Prevention, the New York State Department of Health, and New York State Department of Environmental Conservation Police, as well as Nassau and Suffolk Counties, for joining efforts with the city's Department of Health to assist the Queens community in taking all the necessary precautions.

"In addition to the confirmed cases including the fatality which occurred this week, DOH is investigating one other death and 24 possible cases primarily from this area of Queens of other individuals. . . ."

PRESS RELEASE

New York City Department of Health Office of Public Affairs

IMMEDIATE RELEASE: Friday, September 24, 1999

THE U.S. CENTERS FOR DISEASE CONTROL ANNOUNCES THAT BIRDS COLLECTED IN NEW YORK CITY TEST POSITIVE FOR WEST NILE–LIKE VIRUS

Today, the U.S. Centers For Disease Control and Prevention (CDC) informed the New York City and New York State Departments of Health, as well as health officials from neighboring New York counties and the states of New Jersey and Connecticut, that a West Nile–like virus was identified in several bird specimens submitted by the Bronx Zoo, as well as by Westchester County.

West Nile virus is an arbovirus closely related to St. Louis Encephalitis (SLE), but it generally causes a milder disease in humans. Both viruses are transmitted through the bite of a mosquito that becomes infected by feeding on an infected bird. Like SLE, West Nile virus is not transmitted person-to-person or from birds to persons. West Nile virus has never before been identified in the United States or any other area of the Western Hemisphere.

Health Commissioner Neal L. Cohen, M.D., said: "Health officials at the New York City DOH, the New York State DOH, and the CDC are currently investigating whether there is any association between these findings and the confirmed SLE cases among people from New York City and Westchester County." In conjunction with the CDC and surrounding states and counties, DOH is also actively investigating whether the deaths of a number of crows in New York City this summer are related to the West Nile–like virus. "Our proactive efforts taken over the past three weeks to control the mosquito population and to advise New Yorkers to take precautions against mosquito bites were appropriate measures to have taken against any mosquito-borne virus," Dr. Cohen concluded.

CDC officials said they will perform additional laboratory tests to determine if patients who were diagnosed with SLE, or who had encephalitis symptoms but whose illnesses were not confirmed as SLE, were related to the West Nile–like virus.

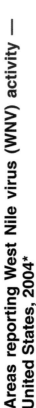

Areas reporting West Nile virus (WNV) activity — United States, 2004*

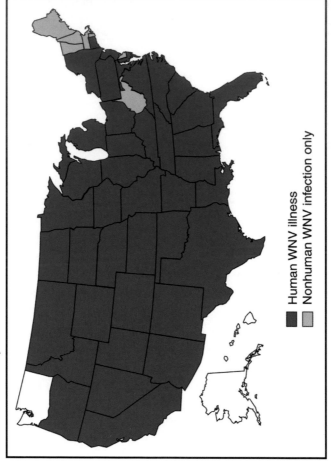

Human WNV illness

Nonhuman WNV infection only

* As of 3 A.M., Mountain Standard Time, November 16, 2004.

Figure 1.1 A map of the United States from the Centers for Disease Control and Prevention shows the distribution of West Nile Virus, a virus that can cause encephalitis, as of November, 2004. Since the first known U.S. cases were identified in 1999, this map illustrates that a virus can spread across a continent relatively quickly, and along with it the risk of encephalitis.

(continued from page 9)

kinds of viruses that most often cause encephalitis are listed in Table 1.1. Nonviral causes of encephalitis, are listed in Table 1.2. In the United States, most cases of encephalitis are caused by viruses such as herpes simplex viruses 1 and 2, rabies, or the class of viruses to which West Nile belongs, referred to as flaviviruses. (*Flavus* means "yellow" in Latin, and the name comes from the first virus discovered in that family: yellow fever virus.) The life cycle and **epidemiology** (the conditions and factors that influence whether a disease or pathogen is present or absent at a particular time and place) of different kinds of viruses that cause encephalitis will be discussed in Chapter 6.

Before we get into too much detail, what exactly are viruses? The word *virus* comes from the Latin word for "poison." Viruses are parasites. As you probably know, a **parasite** is an organism that gets its essential nutrition from other living organisms. Viruses must live inside the cells of organisms and cannot replicate (reproduce) on their own. They are therefore referred to as *obligate parasites*. Almost every kind of living organism, from bacteria to humans, can be infected by some kind of virus. However, not all viral infections produce symptoms or disease.

The existence of viruses has been recognized for a long time, long before their molecular nature was understood. People living in ancient Egypt around 3700 B.C. recorded diseases that were caused by viruses. In 1909, poliomyelitis (better known as "polio") became the first human disease that scientists could prove was caused directly by a virus. This book is written almost a century later, at a time when many seriously debilitating symptoms and diseases are now known to originate from viral infections.

This book attempts to shed some light on the general aspects of one such disease: encephalitis. You will learn about the biological basis of this disease, including some information about viruses, the immune system, the nervous system, and

(continued on page 16)

Table 1.1 Viruses That Cause Encephalitis

Adenoviruses, which also cause respiratory infections
Colorado tick virus, which also causes Colorado tick fever
Cytomegalovirus, which also causes a common childhood infection with mild symptoms
Enteroviruses, which also cause poliomyelitis and often cause upper respiratory infections
Epstein-Barr virus, which also causes mononucleosis
European and Far Eastern (Russian) encephalitis virus, which are spread by ticks
Herpes simplex viruses, the viruses that also cause cold sores and genital herpes
Human immunodeficiency virus (HIV), the virus that causes AIDS
Japanese encephalitis, which is spread by mosquitoes
La Crosse encephalitis virus
Measles virus, which also causes measles
Rubella virus, which also causes German measles
St. Louis encephalitis virus
Varicella zoster viruses, which also cause shingles and chicken pox
Western and Eastern equine encephalitis virus
West Nile virus

Table 1.2 Nonviral Causes of Encephalitis

BACTERIA
Bartonella henselae
Bartonella quintana
Borrelia burgdorferi
Brucella species
Leptospira interrogans
Listeria monocytogenes
Mycobacterium tuberculosis
Mycoplasma pneumoniae
Rickettsia rickettsii
Treponema pallidum
Bacterial infection within the brain
Partially treated bacterial meningitis
PROTOZOA
Naegleria fowleri
Acanthamoeba species
Cysticercosis
Echinococcus species
Plasmodium falciparum
Trypanosoma species
FUNGI
Blastomycosis
Coccidioidomycosis
Cryptococcosis
Histoplasmosis

(continued from page 13)

how the interaction of all three can result in encephalitis. You will also learn about the different kinds of viruses that cause encephalitis. The symptoms, methods of diagnosis, treatment, and prevention of encephalitis are also explored. There is a discussion of the importance of the roles local, state, federal, and global public health organizations have in monitoring and responding to all infectious disease outbreaks. Finally, the last chapter presents some insight into ongoing scientific research and the possibilities for public health measures to treat encephalitis in the future.

2

Viruses: The Molecular Basis for Encephalitis

Encephalitis is a term used to describe an acute inflammation of the brain. It is not actually a disease in and of itself, but a condition caused by another infection. The most common underlying cause of encephalitis is infection by a virus. Therefore, it is important to understand what a virus is, how it infects human cells, and how a viral infection can enter the nervous system.

As you read in Chapter 1, it was only about 100 years ago that scientists first defined what a virus is. At the time, experts thought viruses were simply biological agents that could pass through a filter too small for bacteria but that were able to transmit diseases to other organisms, such as plants and animals. Today, we know that not all viruses are smaller than all bacteria. And it is unclear if we should consider viruses living things, like bacteria are. Viruses are most commonly defined as submicroscopic organisms that are *obligate intracellular parasites*, which means that they must live inside a **host** cell to survive.

Viruses do not "grow" in the traditional way—through the cell division process that many biological organisms use to reproduce. Instead, viruses "replicate," or copy, themselves. To do so, they hijack the molecular machinery of a host cell and force it to manufacture viral components instead of performing its usual function. Then, the viruses take these components and assemble them into many copies of themselves. In this way, the number of viruses is multiplied many times within a single host cell. This strategy has worked well thus far—the number of viruses that exist on Earth is enormous—there are estimated to be 10^{30} virus particles in the oceans alone! (A trillion is 10^{12}, and the word for 10^{30} is "nonillion.")

MOLECULAR ANATOMY OF A VIRUS

The genetic information of viruses and all living organisms is enclosed in chains of molecules called DNA and RNA. Polymers, a linked series of small molecules, called either **deoxyribonucleic acid** (**DNA**) or **ribonucleic acid** (**RNA**), are thought to contain the genetic information of all living organisms, including viruses. DNA and RNA are both made up of small subunits, called **nucleotides**, that incorporate a sugar, a base, and a small chemical entity called a phosphate group. DNA and RNA differ in the kind of sugar they use and also have some structural differences. In both cases, nucleotides are linked together side by side to form a polymer, which is often referred to as a "strand" (Figure 2.1). Although there are some exceptions, DNA is usually double-stranded, which means that two parallel strands are linked together. RNA, on the other hand, is usually single-stranded. These DNA and RNA strands encode for all of the proteins found within the cell. (A strand of DNA that encodes for a single protein is called a "gene.") In order to create the protein, the genetic material undergoes a series of reactions that follow a predictable pathway. First, the DNA sequence is transcribed (rewritten) into messenger RNA (mRNA). Then, the mRNA sequence is translated into protein. This information flow from DNA to mRNA to protein is called the **central dogma** of modern biology. However, it turns out that certain viruses, such as West Nile virus, sometimes reverse the process and instead use an RNA **genome** to encode their DNA. In fact, there are also some viruses that never use DNA at all and go straight from RNA translation into the cytoplasm of the infected cell.

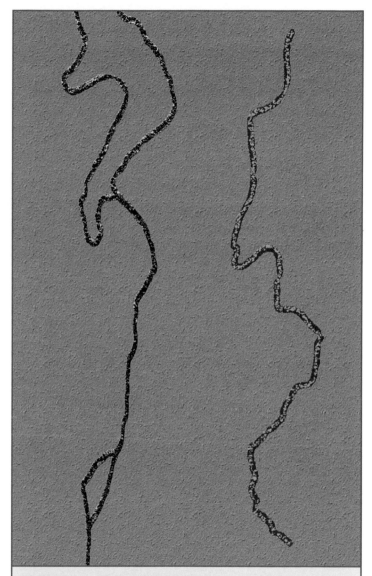

Figure 2.1 An image taken with a transmission electron microscope (X20,000 magnification) of a "strand" of DNA (on left) and a "strand" of RNA (on right). The "strands" are really polymers that are formed by nucleotides that are linked side by side. DNA is usually double stranded and RNA is usually single stranded.

Regardless of whether it is made up of DNA or RNA, a genome refers to all of the genetic information of a particular organism. Viruses are divided into groups based on the type of genome they have. Genetically speaking, viruses are able to "pack lightly." They only carry a relatively small quantity of essential genetic information with them. Therefore, at its smallest, a viral genome can contain just a few genes. By comparison, the human genome consists of approximately 30,000 genes, while a common bacterium, *Escherichia coli*, has about 4,000 genes. The complete genomes of many organisms, including several viruses that can cause encephalitis, are now known.

In general, a viral genome is encased by a coat of proteins, which helps minimize damage from potential hazards, such as the ultraviolet (UV) rays of the sun. The most basic viral coat is called a **capsid** and is made of clusters of proteins referred to as **capsomers**. The capsid is what gives viruses their characteristic shape. The term **nucleocapsid** refers to both the genetic core and the surrounding capsid. In addition to protecting the genome, the capsid also helps the virus infect a host cell by acting as a courier, delivering the viral genome into the host cell. The capsid does this either by forming a **pore** or channel through the membrane of the cell through which the genetic material is injected. Alternatively, the entire virus can be internalized into the cell through endocytosis. Following entry, the virus breaks up the organelles and hijacks the host cell machinery to transcribe it genome. The capsid may or may not be wrapped up in another layer of protection, an **envelope** made of proteins and lipids. **Lipids,** (from the Greek word for "fat," *lipos*) are water-insoluble, carbon-based (organic) molecules that are the major ingredients of all cellular membranes. Some examples of lipids are fats, waxes, and steroids. The viral envelope helps viruses attach to host cells and in certain types of viruses, proteins in the envelope can help the virus merge with the surface of the cell and get inside it. In other types of enveloped viruses, proteins in the envelope can

(continued on page 23)

THE HUMAN GENOME PROJECT

In the mid-1980s, technological advances made it possible to auto-mate the process of determining the exact order of nucleotides in a piece of DNA or RNA, referred to as "genome sequencing." This prompted a small group of scientists to propose a very large and expensive experiment: to sequence the entire human genome. At the time, the human genome was estimated to contain approximately 100,000 different genes. By comparison, in 1984, scientists accomplished the first complete genome sequencing—that of the Epstein-Barr virus—which was thought to be 20,000 times smaller. (As you will read below, it turned out that the human genome is much smaller than most scientists expected.)

Despite the ambitiousness of the experiment and skepticism from much of the scientific community, a consortium of scientists from the U.S. Department of Energy, the National Research Council, the National Institutes of Health, and a private nonprofit institute, The Institute for Genomic Research (TIGR), decided to go for it. They also planned to sequence the genomes of other smaller organisms, starting with animals that are useful to scientific research and pathogens that are hazardous to human health. Before the human genome was sequenced, scientists sequenced the genomes of some smaller organisms, starting with those that have the smallest number of genes: Epstein-Barr virus (1984), *H. influenzae* (1995), the yeast *C. cerevisiae* (1996), the bacterium *Escherichia coli* (1997), the worm *C. elegans* (1998), the plant *A. sthaliana* (2000), and the fruit fly *D. melanogaster* (2000). Of all these organisms, *A. sthaliana* had the largest number of genes, at 25,000.

In 1990, the Human Genome Project (HGP) officially began as a publicly funded, coordinated, and international effort. The HGP used an established method of sequencing that was based on put-ting pieces of the human genome into bacteria, sequencing the pieces from the bacteria, and then assembling the sequences one at a time using what was already known about how genes are organized. Starting in 1998, a private company, Celera Genomics, began using a different approach, called whole-genome shotgun sequencing, to try to sequence the human genome. This method broke the human genome up into random short overlapping pieces and then assembled the sequence all at once using new computer software.

In the same week of February 2001, the two scientific teams published their preliminary results in two leading international scientific journals, *Nature* (Human Genome Project) and *Science* (Celera Genomics). The articles were entitled "Initial Sequencing and Analysis of the Human Genome" and "The Sequencing of the Human Genome," respectively. Surprisingly, both groups concluded that the total number of human genes is a lot smaller than had previously been thought. Instead of 100,000 human genes, there are only about 30,000. In order to account for the diversity of biological material in human cells, it seems that these 30,000 genes are rearranged in a multitude of ways, kind of like rearranging the same set of words to make a different sentence.

As already mentioned, the genomes of organisms used routinely in scientific research, such as various worms, fruit flies, bacteria, and viruses have been sequenced. This information helps researchers understand how genetic mutations can cause or lend susceptibility to certain human diseases. Furthermore, the sequencing of different genomes allows researchers to study how basic biological processes in different organisms are related. Recently, scientists began sequencing a whole new population of previously unknown organisms that live in the Sargasso Sea near Bermuda. They have already found 1.2 million new genes, some of them encoding members of protein families that play important functions in human biology such as receptors for light. Comparing different organisms, such as a mouse and a man, often reveals which steps in a biological process are vital and which ones are more specialized or optional. Or, they can reveal a completely different mechanism altogether that accomplishes the same thing. All of these studies are useful to the discovery of new ways to treat and prevent human disease.

(continued from page 20)

merge with membranes inside the cell, gaining access to the machinery of the cell that the virus needs to reproduce itself. West Nile virus, as well as some of the other viruses that can cause encephalitis, are enveloped. Based on their type of genome, capsid proteins, and envelope, viruses can come in many different shapes and sizes (Figure 2.2).

THE INITIAL STAGES OF VIRAL INFECTION

So how does a virus actually enter a cell? Just as a thief with a copied key can open a lock that is not his, a virus begins to enter a cell via a similar type of crime. The outermost layer of a virus has special proteins that latch onto a cell and "pick" the molecular locks on its surface. These locks, which cover the surface of a cell, are called **receptors**. When there is no virus attached to the cell, receptors are used to convey important signals from the outside world to the inside of the cell. Unrelated viruses can attach (**bind**) at different times to the same kind of receptor on a cell surface. Many molecules can bind with multiple kinds of molecular partners, so the same receptor may "fit" several different types of viruses. In general, viruses bind to cell surface receptors that are either common (easy to come by) or particular to a certain kind of cell. For example, the rabies virus, which can cause encephalitis, binds to receptors that are mainly found only on nerve cells (neurons). A virus's preference for infecting a certain type of cell (like a neuron) is called **tropism**, and is caused by the specific interaction of the virus with a receptor found on that kind of cell.

In addition to binding to a cell surface receptor, a virus often has to bind to a second cell surface receptor, called a **co-receptor**. In these cases, it is only after this second inter-action that a virus can enter into a cell.

An example of a virus that can cause encephalitis and needs a co-receptor to infect is the human immunodeficiency virus (HIV), the virus that causes acquired immunodeficiency syndrome (AIDS). Strains of this virus interact with receptors

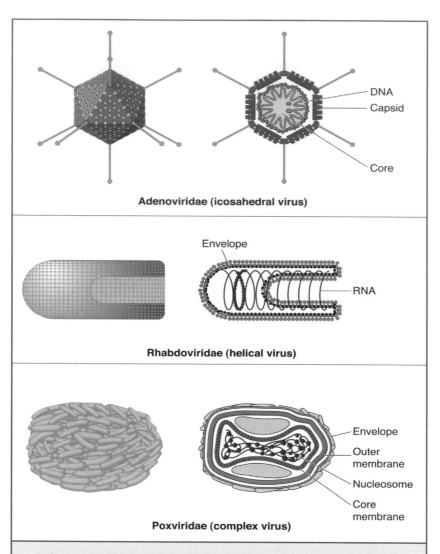

Figure 2.2 Viruses come in different shapes and sizes. A schematic illustration shows three different viruses. One of the smallest DNA viruses is shown in the upper panel. In the center of the virus is the nucleic acid core, surrounded by a coating of proteins called the capsid. In the middle panel is an example of an RNA virus that has an outer envelope. In the lower panel is a larger virus that has an outer membrane of protection in addition to the envelope. Viruses in each of these families can cause encephalitis.

and co-receptors that are expressed on certain types of white blood cells that play critical roles in fighting **microbial** infections. That is why HIV is particularly debilitating to the immune system—the virus targets the kind of cells that would normally help the host fight off an infection. Interestingly, scientists have discovered the molecular explanation for why a small number of people exposed to HIV do not become infected with the virus. The reason is that these people have a change (**mutation**) in the gene for an HIV co-receptor, and therefore make a form of the co-receptor to which the virus cannot attach. If a virus encounters a cell that does not have the specific receptor or co-receptor to which it can attach, then in most cases, that cell is protected from infection by that particular virus.

VIRAL ENTRY INTO AND EXIT FROM A CELL

After binding to the host cell, different kinds of viruses enter the cell using a variety of strategies. An enveloped virus enters the cell either by blending its envelope together with the **cell membrane** of the host, a process called **fusion**, or by being swallowed up by the cell membrane, a process called **endocytosis**. Viruses that don't have envelopes can bind to a receptor on the surface of the cell. This attachment to the cell surface causes a three-dimensional change in the shape of the viral particle. This change in shape allows a viral capsid protein to poke a hole into the cell, forming a pore through which the rest of the virus can get into the cell. The other way by which non-enveloped viruses can get into cells is by getting swallowed up by endocytosis. In this process, a virus interacts with a receptor that triggers the cell to take the virus inside it. Once the virus is inside the cell, the capsid of the virus binds to the cell's nucleus and releases its genome through a pore that is normally used by the cell to import and export things into and out of the nucleus. Then, the virus hijacks the necessary equipment from the infected cell to replicate its genome (Figure 2.3).

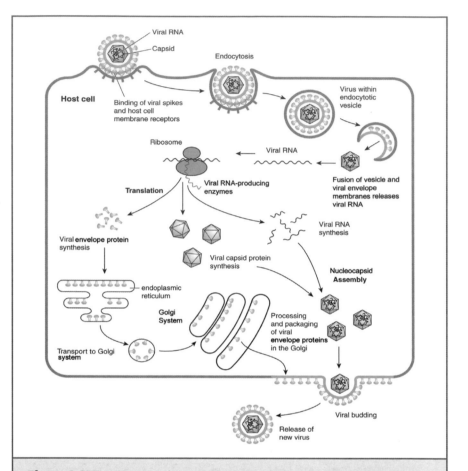

Figure 2.3 The life cycle of an enveloped virus. Not all viruses live identically to the one shown here, but here is an example of the life cycle of an enveloped virus, many of which can cause encephalitis. Proteins on the outer coat of the virus bind to receptors on the cell surface. Through a regulated process called endocytosis, the membrane around the virus pinches off and carries the virus into the cell. This membrane-bound compartment is now called a vesicle. The viral envelope then fuses with the vesicle membrane and releases viral RNA into the cell cytoplasm. The virus then uses the cell's own machinery to transcribe its own RNA to make viral products. The viral RNA is translated into the products needed to make more viral particles—e.g., envelope and capsid proteins. At the same time, more viral RNA is made. The nucleocapsids are assembled and packaged together with other viral products to make new virus particles. Viruses then bud from the membrane and get released into the extracellular space—ready to invade even more cells!

Having accomplished its entry into the cell, the virus uses the host cell to decode its genome and make its own viral proteins. So what, exactly, do most viruses "pack" with them as they travel, looking for a host to infect? In general, viral genomes encode three types of proteins: (1) proteins needed to copy the viral genome; (2) proteins needed to wrap up, or package, and deliver the viral genome; and (3) proteins that exploit the host cell to help the virus survive, including the blueprints for any machinery needed for making the two other kinds of proteins (1) and (2). This **parasitic** lifestyle makes viruses especially challenging for medical professionals to treat because drugs targeted to kill a virus may also inadvertently interfere with some of the normal functions of the infected host cell. That is why, as we will discuss in Chapter 7, public health officials place so much emphasis on the prevention of viral infections.

Once the viral genome has been incorporated as part of the host, the virus uses the host cell to make its own viral proteins, and the ingredients needed to create a new virus particle, called a **virion**, are put together. One virion infecting one host cell can make thousands of copies of itself. Virions then undergo a process of maturation inside the cell, making whatever changes are needed to get them ready to leave the cell and find more hosts for their increased number. Exiting a cell usually occurs in one of two ways. If the virus is non-enveloped, it has limited options for gaining access into another cell, so it often replicates enough virus particles, to cause the infected cell to burst open (**lyse**). This not only kills the host cell but also makes it easy for the virus to spread to new cells within the same organism.

Enveloped viruses use a different method of escape: They acquire a disguise on their way out of the infected host cell. In this case, during the process of leaving the host cell, called *budding*, a virus can wrap itself up in a layer from the outer membrane of the host cell, giving it a way to exit the cell without killing it (Figure 2.4). This kind of virus can sometimes

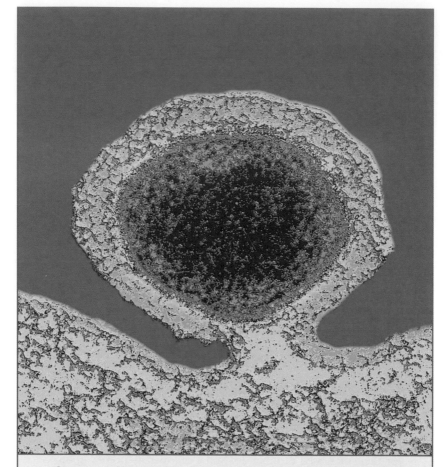

Figure 2.4 Virus budding! A photograph taken by a high powered microscope of an animal cell from which a virus is budding off.

reside in the body for long periods of time and is thought to contribute to the development of certain types of cancers as well as other diseases, including encephalitis.

LATENT VIRAL INFECTIONS

As previously mentioned, some viruses can exist in the body for long periods of time, not actively replicating, but existing instead in a kind of "hibernation." This phase is called **latency**.

Latent viral infections can be very dangerous to the central nervous system (CNS). Normally, pathogens or cells infected by a virus or other pathogen generate proteins, lipids, and carbohydrates that the pathogen needs to survive or proliferate. Pieces of these molecules, called **antigens**, can be detected by the immune system, which can then destroy the offending organism or infected cell. A **latent** viral infection, however, sets itself up in some part of the body and then enters a kind of dormant stage where it stops making any detectable viral products. A latent viral infection can therefore last for a lifetime without ever being seen by the immune system. After various kinds of stimuli, such as stress, another kind of infection, sunlight, or changes in hormone levels, the virus can be re-activated, begin to replicate, and start another round of infection.

Herpes simplex virus-1 (HSV-1) is an example of a virus that can enter latency and can also cause encephalitis. HSV-1 is an extremely common virus that infects 50–90% of adults in all human populations tested. (A closely related virus called herpes simplex virus-2 is usually sexually transmitted and is present in approximately 10% of the adult population.) HSV-1 often infects skin cells, usually of the face. Infected skin cells can become part of a lesion, which can rupture to become cold sores. Most of the virus within the lesion has been killed by the immune system, but some live virus particles can escape.

The renegade virus particles can enter branches of a sensory nerve called the **trigeminal nerve** that serves the areas around the mouth, nose, and eyes. The virus can then hide out in nerve cells without replicating or making any detectable viral products, escaping detection by the immune system as mentioned above. After the infection is reactivated by outside stimuli such as stress, hormonal changes, sunlight, or infection by some other organism, the virus can travel back down the nerve to infect new skin cells. New cold sores are then formed in the same place as the original infection or near the old ones, which may still contain infectious virus. The virus can then spread further into the central nervous system and establish an infection there. This CNS infection can later go on to cause encephalitis.

If you have ever suffered from the terribly itchy and common childhood disease chicken pox, then you have experienced another kind of herpes virus that can enter latency and

MICROORGANISM GENOME PROJECTS

Since the beginning of the Human Genome Project, researchers as well as the general public have realized how valuable it is to know the entire genome sequence of any given organism. Knowledge is power! This is especially true when dealing with pathogens. Therefore, many different U.S. government organizations, including the National Institutes of Health, the Department of Defense, the Centers for Disease Control and Prevention (CDC), and the Department of Homeland Security, are funding projects to sequence and study various strains of microorganisms. Furthermore, reflecting the philosophical value that scientific knowledge is for the benefit of all humankind, and the practical consideration that microbes are the globetrotters on Earth, scientific studies often involve researchers and their governments collaborating from all over the world. With these efforts, the genomes of many viruses that can cause encephalitis have been sequenced. For example, in 2002, researchers from the CDC, working with scientists at the Pasteur Institute in France, determined the complete genome sequence of West Nile virus. Researchers are using viral genomes to study how viruses enter and exit cells, replicate, enter latent states, and, in general, interact with their human hosts. These studies help us understand how viruses may become resistant to drugs or how they escape from the immune system, so that scientists can develop better methods of prevention and treatment.

infect neurons. After the symptoms have subsided, varicella zoster virus, which is the scientific name of the chicken pox virus, can hide out in sensory nerve cells that serve different areas of the skin. Years later, stress or other factors can reactivate the virus, allowing it to spread down the nerves and reinfect the skin cells. When this happens, a rash appears, which is referred to as "shingles." Unlike HSV-1, reactivation of varicella zoster virus usually happens only once in a lifetime. In 2001, scientists in Finland published a study that suggested that the chicken pox virus might actually contribute to more cases of nervous system infections than was previously realized.

3

The Immune System and Viral Infections

You just read about how viruses infect cells and what they do once inside them—replicate! But the majority of patients with viral infections never develop symptoms of encephalitis. The reason for this is that a patient's own immune system is usually able to successfully contain and destroy the virus. How does it do this? To understand the causes (**etiology**) of encephalitis, you need some basic knowledge of both the human immune system and the site of viral infection that relates to encephalitis: the nervous system. This chapter examines the immune system, which is responsible for the inflammation of any tissue, including that of the nervous system, and how it attempts to fight off infections. Chapter 4 will look at what happens when the immune system fails and a virus manages to infect the central nervous system (CNS), which consists of the brain and spinal cord causing encephalitis.

The symptoms of any viral infection are influenced by the route of the infection, the type of cells infected, and consequently, by the patient's own immune response to the infection. Viruses can infect neurons directly (as the rabies virus does), or indirectly (like HIV-1) by first infecting other kinds of cells that may migrate into the central nervous system, or through a combination of the two routes. Once in a nerve cell, a virus can multiply within it, killing the cell in the process. Tropism (as mentioned in Chapter 2) refers to what kinds of cells a virus specifically targets to invade. This concept is particularly crucial in the CNS, since it influences which areas of the brain are most affected.

Because most nerve cells are long-lived, not easily replaced, and may be connected to more than one other nerve cell, any damage to them can have long-lasting effects on the patient. Most viral infections start somewhere else in the body other than the CNS. So how do they gain access to the nervous system? The answer is that viral infections commonly lead to **inflammation**, a process described below, which can produce conditions that allow a virus to enter to the CNS.

OVERVIEW OF THE IMMUNE SYSTEM

Although different viruses are more or less prevalent among different demographic groups, the people most at risk for developing encephalitis are the immunocompromised (people who have a weakened immune system). This state can be due to a number of different underlying causes, such as age (the immune system tends to weaken as we get older), other diseases like diabetes or AIDS, infection by another pathogen, or even some medications, such as those used to treat cancer. The next sections explain the basic strategies that the immune system uses to fight viral infections and what may happen when a virus overwhelms it and enters the CNS.

There are two types of immune responses: innate and adaptive. We have our innate immune response from the time we are born. It is preprogrammed to recognize certain features of pathogens. The **adaptive immune response** develops throughout our lives and has an infinite ability to change, expand, and remember the microbes we encounter. All animals—even fruit flies and worms—have an **innate immune system**, but only vertebrates (animals with spinal cords and a separate brain) also have an **adaptive immune system**. All cells of the immune system, collectively referred to as **white blood cells**, or **leukocytes**, develop in the bone marrow from blood **stem cells** (Figure 3.1). White blood cells migrate from the bone marrow to sites throughout the body, where they guard against pathogens. White blood cells are important players in every

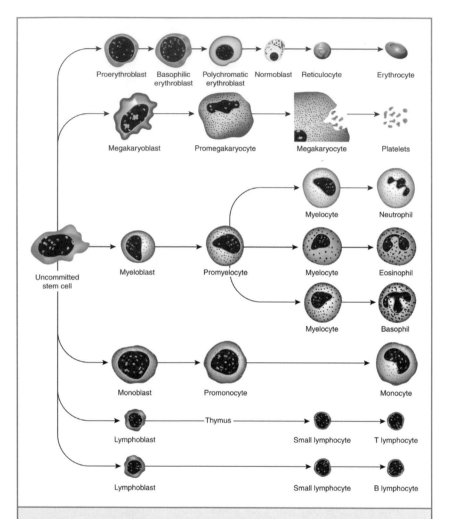

Figure 3.1 All blood cells arise from a stem cell. An undifferentiated stem cell in the bone marrow gives rise to all of the different cell types of the immune system. An erythrocyte is a red blood cell. Platelets are crucial for blood clotting. Neutrophils are critical during inflammation. Eosinophils are particularly important in parasitic infections. Basophils are important during allergic reactions. Monocytes give rise to macrophages, the most phagocytic of immune cells, which are very important to innate immunity. T lymphocytes mature in the thymus and are responsible for cell-mediated immunity. B cells are responsible for humoral immunity and make all of the antibodies in your body.

step of viral encephalitis, from fighting the infection to reducing the inflammation of the nervous system and the subsequent recovery of the host. The cells of the immune system and their chemical products are even used to aid in figuring out which kind of viral infection encephalitis patients have, as will be described in Chapter 5.

Before we examine innate immunity, we should briefly discuss another kind of cell that is responsible for staving off lots of potential infections—epithelial cells. **Epithelial** cells make up the skin and line the respiratory, gastrointestinal, and genital tracts. Simply put, epithelial cells protect your insides from what is outside. They do not form just a passive physical barrier, either—**epithelia** (the singular form is *epithelium*) in different locations actively make a number of antimicrobial substances that help kill potentially infectious organisms. That is why a mosquito or animal bite is such a great way for a virus to enter the body—it gets the virus across the first immune barrier and right into the blood!

The Innate Immune System

During the first hours and days following the start of an infection, the innate immune system uses some general mechanisms to try to eliminate the pathogen. Using special receptors that detect molecular ingredients common to different microorganisms, white blood cells called **macrophages** (from the Greek words meaning "large eater") and **neutrophils**, which are also good at eating and killing pathogens, try to identify the pathogen and destroy it, sometimes calling on other types of cells for help. To accomplish these tasks, macrophages and neutrophils eat and drink from the area surrounding infected cells and thereby ingest chemical products or even tiny pieces of the pathogen itself that they can later show to other immune system cells. The process of engulfing the organism is called **phagocytosis**, and drinking the fluid around the infected cells is called "pinocytosis."

Once they have gobbled up a pathogen, macrophages and neutrophils can then destroy it.

Another cell type, called **natural killer (NK) cells**, can specifically recognize cells that are infected with viruses. They do this by "asking" a cell for a kind of "secret handshake." What does this mean at the molecular level? Almost all healthy cells flag their surfaces with a particular protein that lets the rest of the body know that it is part of the body—a "self" cell. This "healthy cell" protein is called **major histocompatibility complex** class I (MHCI). NK cells have proteins that normally interact with MHCI, called killer-cell inhibitory receptors (KIR). When an NK cell bumps into another cell, it waits for its KIR to be met with MHCI. If it is not, the NK cell knows that something is wrong and releases molecules that are **cytotoxic** (*cyto* means "cell" and *toxic* means "poison" or "lethal") and kills the other cell. It just so happens that many virally infected cells have less MHCI on their surface, giving NK cells an opportunity to detect and kill them. Interestingly, for this reason, NK cells are able to kill some tumor cells.

There are also proteins called **complement** that circulate in the blood. These proteins stick to the outer surfaces of pathogens, such as the envelopes of some viruses, tagging them so that they can be identified and removed by macrophages.

Inflammation

Inflammation is a process that begins when there is damage to a body tissue. This damage can come from almost any cause, including mechanical injury like breaking a bone, or an infection by a pathogen. In the inflammation process, the immune system works toward three goals: sending in cells to kill the invading organism, cordoning off the infected area so the pathogen does not spread further, and repairing the damage that has already been done. Early in their education, every medical student learns to characterize inflammation by four Latin words, first used by a physician named Celsus during the days of the

Roman Empire: *dolor* (pain), *tumor* (swelling), *calor* (heat), and *rubor* (redness). During the last 2,000 years, physicians and scientists have begun to unravel some of the molecular changes that cause these obvious signs of inflammation.

One of the first cell types to be engaged in the process of inflammation is the macrophage. As soon as macrophages detect a pathogen, they begin to release chemical signals called **cytokines** and **chemokines**. Cytokines sent from one cell bind to other cells that have a matching sensor (receptor) for them, triggering profound molecular changes in the cells that receive them, such as changes in the genes they are making. One early defensive measure by white blood cells is the production of a class of anti-viral cytokines called **interferons**—named for their ability to "interfere" with the process of viral replication. These molecules have been shown to be important in influencing susceptibility to West Nile and other viral infections. Cells infected with viruses produce interferons and release them into

(continued on page 40)

NOBEL PRIZES FOR WORK WITH VIRUSES AND THE IMMUNE SYSTEM

In 1900, a foundation was established under the terms of the will of Alfred Nobel, a Swedish man who invented dynamite in the 19th century. Through the Nobel Foundation, a prize is given annually in the fields of physics, chemistry, physiology or medicine, literature, and peace. The Bank of Sweden awards a prize in economic sciences in memory of Alfred Nobel, which is accorded the same prestige as a Nobel Prize, even though it is technically not one. The amount of each prize is approximately $1 million and can be shared by up to three scientists in each category per year. If it is shared, it is usually among people who made related discoveries. Table 3.1 shows the scientists who have won Nobel Prizes for their work on issues that relate to viruses (the most common cause of encephalitis).

Table 3.1 Adapted from a chronology of discoveries and the scientists who made them

YEAR	NAME(S)	DISCOVERY (VIRUS GROUP OR FAMILY)
1999	Stanley B. Prusiner	Discovery of prions, a new infectious agent
1996	Rolf M. Zinkernagel Peter C. Doherty	How the immune system recognizes virus-infected cells
1993	Phillip A. Sharp Richard J. Roberts	Discovery that genes can split themselves, using the virus that causes the common cold (*Adenoviridae*)
1989	J. Michael Bishop Harold E. Varmus	Discovery of the cellular origin of retroviral oncogenes, genes that help control the growth and division of cells and can go awry in cancer
1988	George H. Hitchings Gertrude B. Elion	New principles of drug development based on differences in metabolism of different organisms, including antiviral drugs called acyclovir (the first drug available to treat herpes virus infections)
1982	Aaron Klug	Development of a new way to look at biological material using X rays, called crystallographic electron microscopy, which showed the structure of many viruses (*Tobamovirus* and *Tymovirus*)
1980	Paul Berg	Studies of nucleic acids; making synthetic DNA using a virus called SV40 (*Polyomaviridae*) that infects apes

1978	Daniel Nathans	Helped invent a biological way to cut DNA with molecules called restriction enzymes, using a virus that infects apes called SV40 (*Polyomaviridae*)
1976	Daniel Carleton Gajdusek Baruch S. Blumberg	Discovery of the cause of kuru, a disease caused by an infectious substance called a prion, and discovery of hepatitis B virus that chronically infects more than 100 million people worldwide
1975	David Baltimore Howard M. Temin Renato Dulbecco	Discoveries concerning interactions between tumor viruses and the cell *(Retroviridae)*
1969	Max Delbrück Alfred D. Hershey Salvador Luria	How viruses infect cells; viruses that infect bacteria (called bacteriophages)
1966	Francis Peyton Rous	Discovery of tumor-causing viruses *(Retroviridae)*
1965	François Jacob André Lwoff Jacques Monod	Discovery of genetic control of enzyme and viral synthesis
1958	Joshua Lederberg	Discovery of genetic recombination and organization of bacteria; and bacteriophages
1954	John F. Enders Thomas H. Weller Frederick C. Robbins	Discovery of how to grow poliovirus in the laboratory and in a variety of tissues *(Picornaviridae)*
1951	Max Theiler	Development of yellow fever virus vaccine (*Flaviviridae*)
1946	Wendell M. Stanley	Isolation, purification, and structure of the tobacco mosaic virus (*Tobamovirus*)

(continued from page 37)

the surrounding area. Other cells bind with these molecules, which tell them to begin a genetic antiviral defense program. Interferons also help start the adaptive immune response.

Rubor (redness) and *calor* (heat) occur because white blood cells produce cytokines and other "**acute phase proteins**" that help cause an inflammation. These factors cause changes in cells that line and make up blood vessels, called endothelial cells. Locally, blood flow increases, then the diameter of blood vessels increases, decreasing the rate of blood flow, and the vessel walls become sticky. This allows white blood cells to attach to and cross the vessel, gaining access to the affected area. Chemokines help further direct cellular traffic to the infection site through the blood vessels, so that other cells can pour into the affected region and help fight the infection. This influx of white blood cells and fluid can cause *dolor* (pain) and *tumor* (swelling). In the process, endothelial cells change shape and move away from each other, allowing the blood vessels (vasculature) to become leaky. At some level, the leaks can be beneficial, allowing more white blood cells and other anti-microbial substances into the area. However, the leak of the local vasculature can also be harmful, because it can help spread a pathogen, such as a virus, into new areas of the body. Taken together, this whole process is referred to as inflammation. In the next chapter you will read that in the case of encephalitis, a very special vasculature, called the **blood-brain barrier**, is often compromised, allowing viruses or virus-infected cells to enter an otherwise healthy central nervous system.

The Adaptive Immune Response

The innate immune response has two major limitations. The first is that it recognizes pathogens based on commonalities rather than on individual features, so it cannot recognize all invaders that may come along. The second limitation is that the innate immune response is on a kind of permanent "reset" mode—it cannot remember what it has encountered before, which leaves the host vulnerable to later infections by the same organism. The adaptive immune response, however, is just that—*adaptive*. It adapts to the substances it meets and can remember the encounter so that the next time it comes across the same substance or organism, it can quickly scale up its response to get rid of it.

How does it do this? Cells of the adaptive immune system, called **lymphocytes**, arise from the same blood stem cells that gives rise to cells of the innate immune system. Lymphocytes mature in primary lymphoid organs, such as the thymus, and bone marrow. Once they are mature, lymphocytes circulate in the blood and tissues. They gather at communication hubs throughout the body, called peripheral lymphoid organs. Examples of such organs include the lymph nodes (which are found throughout the body, including under the armpits and behind the knees), spleen (located in the abdomen), and tonsils (at the back of the throat) (Figure 3.2a). Lymphocytes from an infected area travel via a special transport network called the lymphatic vessels, which drain water and proteins from tissues throughout the body back into the bloodstream. The lymphatic vessels are similar to blood vessels and are often found close to blood vessels. The lymphatic vessels are the route by which fluid from swollen areas gets removed. The draining of fluids through the lymphatics goes through hubs, called lymph nodes (Figure 3.2b). Lymph nodes are where lymphocytes wait to fight off pathogens. By coming into contact with material from a site of infection, lymphocytes can learn about the molecular nature of the offending pathogen and start to adapt the immune response to fight off that particular organism. Have you ever wondered why your health-care provider feels the sides of your neck just below your ears when you come into the office suffering from flu-like symptoms? Well, it's to check for swollen lymph nodes, a clinical sign of infection that occurs because cells and fluid are pouring in from the infected areas through the lymphatic vessels. Swollen lymph

(continued on page 44)

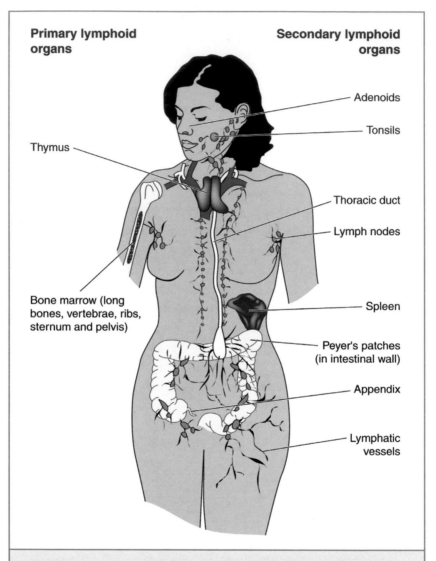

Figure 3.2a The immune system: primary and secondary lymphoid organs. Lymphocytes develop from stem cells in the bone marrow, and differentiate in the central lymphoid organs. **B cells** differentiate in the bone marrow and **T cells** in the thymus. They then travel via the bloodstream to the peripheral or secondary lymphoid organs, which are the lymph nodes, the spleen, and lymphoid tissues associated with mucosa such as the tonsils, Peyer's patches of the intestinal wall, adenoids, and appendix.

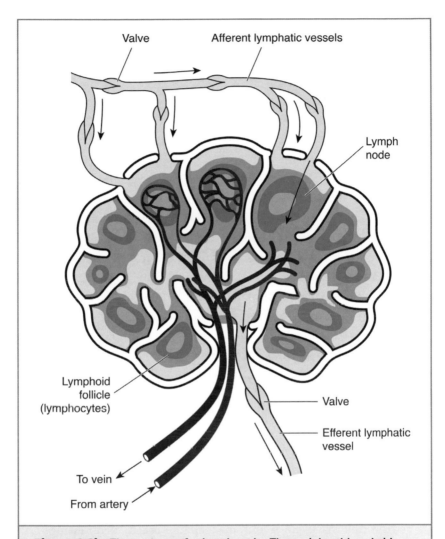

Figure 3.2b The anatomy of a lymph node. The peripheral lymphoid organs are the sites of lymphocyte activation by antigen from pathogens like viruses. Afferent lymphatic vessels drain extracellular fluid from the peripheral tissues through the lymph node, and efferent lymphatic vessels drain finally to a vein. This fluid, known as lymph, carries antigens to the lymph nodes and recirculating immune cells from the lymph nodes back into the blood. Different types of lymphocytes concentrate in different areas of the node where they interact with local cells, instructing them about what antigens they have encountered outside of the lymph nodes.

(continued from page 41)

nodes can occur even in the case of CNS infections because most infections of the CNS first begin outside of the CNS.

Humoral Immunity

B cells, which mature in the bone marrow, are the source of **humoral immunity**, meaning immunity that involves antibodies. Each B cell has a unique protein, called an **antibody**, displayed on its surface. When the antibody binds the molecule it was built to detect, the B cell becomes activated. When it gets the antigen, or confirmation from another cell that something is amiss, the B cell begins to divide and produce identical copies of itself, called **clones**. After about four to five days, the clone replication (expansion) is complete. The clones can then release the same antibody as the original B cell, allowing it to bind to the antigen it recognizes. This binding can sometimes lead to the killing of a microorganism directly or can flag the pathogen to be killed by other cells of the immune system. Some kinds of antibodies can remain in the circulatory system for years or even decades, providing long-lasting protection against such pathogens. When the same substance is encountered again, specific antibody can be increased very quickly to get rid of the invader before it can start an infection. This immunological memory, as you will read in Chapter 7, is the principle behind vaccination.

There are several ways that antibodies can contribute to controlling a viral infection. Some antibodies can bind to a virus and inactivate it and are therefore called "neutralizing antibodies." Other antibodies can bind to a virus and not inactivate it, but still help clear the viral infection. One way antibodies can do this is by acting as a kind of sponge for circulating virus particles, sopping them up and making them unavailable to infect new cells. Antibodies can also bind to pieces of a virus that are complexed with the MHC proteins on the surface of an infected cell, marking the cell to be killed by the immune system. Even in the womb, antibodies are passed from mother to fetus, helping to protect the fetus and newborn against viral infections.

Cell-mediated Immunity

Cell-mediated immunity is directed by T cells, which mature in the thymus. Like snowflakes, no two T cells (or B cells, for that matter) are exactly alike! Each T cell has a unique sensor (receptor) that can detect pieces of an antigen from a micro-organism or a piece of a microbial product. At any given time, a person has cells with more than 100 million different T cell receptors. A kind of checkpoint for T cells with different T cell receptors occurs in the thymus, so that newly made T cells that can recognize material made by the host, and are potentially harmful to the body, are eliminated. Because viruses live and hide inside other cells, substances released from other white blood cells into the circulatory system are ineffective at combating viruses directly. Some T cells, called **cytotoxic T cells** or **killer T cells**, similar to NK cells, can recognize cells infected with viruses and kill them. They do this in a way that is complimentary to NK cells. While NK cells are looking for "self" signals, killer T cells are looking for signs of "nonself." How do they do this? Cells that are infected with viruses (or other pathogens) sometimes flag themselves as infected by wedging a tiny scrap of a viral material, called an antigen, into their MHC molecule, which then gets waved on their surface. This process of waving, or "presenting," a viral anti-gen on the cell surface is called **antigen presentation**. T cells can detect the "flag," recognize cells that have been infected with viruses, and kill them via a process called apoptosis (Figure 3.3).

Another type of T cells is called a **helper T cell**. Helper T cells can also relay information about an infection to other cells in the immune system, such as B cells, to help mount the body's counterattack. They do this, for example, by releasing signaling molecules called cytokines.

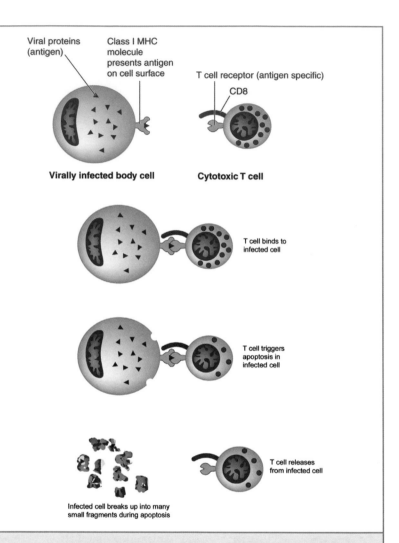

Figure 3.3 Killer T cells get mobilized during a viral infection. Killer T cells express a cell surface molecule called "CD8." A T cell receptor displayed on the surface of the cell is specific for a particular antigen—in this illustration, a viral antigen. When this T cell encounters a cell that has been infected by a virus and displays the same viral antigen on its surface attached to a MHCI molecule, the T cell binds to the infected cell. The T cell then releases factors that trigger a genetic program for "suicide" within the infected cell, called "apoptosis." The infected cell breaks up into many small pieces and the killer T cell releases its attachment to the infected cell.

Other Types of Adaptive Immune Responses

Some cells of the adaptive immune system hang around after the infection is resolved, so that the next time the body comes across the same substance, it can quickly scale up its response to prevent an infection before it starts. These cells are on a kind of "ready alert" state all the time and are able to respond very quickly when the same organism is encountered again, making large amounts of antibodies or lots of specific T cells. This **immunological memory** is critical to the success of blocking infection by viruses with vaccines—a topic that will be covered in Chapter 7.

Initiation of the Immune System: Dendritic Cells

Ironically for students reading about viral encephalitis, the cells most critical to the initiation of the adaptive immune response were actually named for their striking resemblance to neurons. These white blood cells were only discovered in 1973 at The Rockefeller University in New York City by Professors Ralph Steinman and the late Zanvil Cohn. The cells were named **dendritic cells** because they extend long tendrils that looked to the researchers who discovered them like the elongated processes found on nerve cells, called **dendrites**.

Dendritic cells also develop in the bone marrow and then live in an "immature" state in the blood, tissues, skin, and **mucosa** (the mucus-coated lining of organs such as the nose, mouth, lungs, and intestinal tract), and elsewhere throughout the body. Dendritic cells serve as "watchdogs" or "guards" of the immune system, constantly taking in material (via endocytosis) from the environment around them, thus surveying the area. Unlike macrophages, which eat a pathogen and then destroy almost all of the evidence, dendritic cells digest the pathogen much more slowly. Once dendritic cells realize that they have eaten something that does not "agree" with them, they begin to change their behavior dramatically. They decrease their rate of sampling the environment and crawl to the nearest lymph node or peripheral lymphoid organ, where they subsequently "vomit" pieces of the digested pathogen onto their surface to present to the B and T cells. As mentioned earlier, this process is called antigen presentation. Although other cell types such as macrophages can also present antigens to other cells, dendritic cells are known as the most potent of antigen presentation cells. As a result of their interactions with dendritic cells, B cells that recognize the flag make antibodies against the pathogen, and T cells that recognize the flag can clone themselves in order to help fight off the infection. During the last five years or so, scientists have also discovered that dendritic cells can enhance the ability of NK cells to kill their targets. Dendritic cells are particularly important in activating the immune response during any kind of infection, but play a particularly important role in viral infections, because viruses often hide inside other cells and escape detection by many cells of the innate immune system. Unfortunately, viruses that can cause encephalitis, such as HIV-1 and cytomegalovirus, can infect dendritic cells. Fortunately, some viral antigens can get presented on the surface of the infected dendritic cells, flagging them to the surrounding cells. Viral infection of dendritic cells has also been show to disrupt the normal functions of dendritic cells—for example, by making them less efficient at presenting antigens to other cells and changing the profile of cytokines they produce to activate other cells of the immune system.

VIRUSES VERSUS THE IMMUNE SYSTEM

One major limitation of the innate immune system is its ability to combat viruses, the main agents that cause encephalitis, because viruses rarely display the common molecular ingredients detected by the receptors of the innate immune system. That is why dendritic cells, which can present a wide variety of viral antigens to lymphocytes, are so important to viral infections. However, many viruses have also evolved an incredible ability to get around the barriers of the adaptive immune system. For example, herpes simplex virus, which can cause encephalitis, is able to block the action of complement and then block the processing and presentation of its antigens. Many viruses, of which HIV-1 is the most dramatic example, can cause a global immunosuppression of a patient, by directly infecting cells of the immune system, giving other pathogens such as bacteria, an enhanced opportunity to infect the patient. These secondary infections are thus called "opportunistic infections."

In this chapter, you have learned about the major cell types of the immune system and some strategies they use to fight off pathogens such as viruses that can cause encephalitis. Cells of the innate immune system such as macrophages try to eat the pathogen or cells infected with a pathogen and then "digest it to death." Macrophages can also kick off a process called inflammation by releasing cytokines and chemokines into infected tissue. Dendritic cells can activate other cells of the innate and adaptive immune systems. Lymphocytes try to recognize a pathogen more precisely and then kill it directly as cytotoxic T cells do by releasing molecules such as antibodies that can harm the pathogen, or by helping flag a pathogen for destruction by other cells. In the next chapter, you will learn what happens when a virus infects the nervous system—the first step toward a case of viral encephalitis.

4

The Nervous System and Viral Infections: Etiology of Encephalitis

It was a muggy afternoon in late July in Queens, New York. Sam, a retired postal worker who loved tending to his small vegetable garden, decided to take an afternoon nap, since he was feeling a bit strange. In fact, he had a terrible headache and felt weak and feverish. By the next morning, his wife, Nancy, noticed that Sam seemed to be very out of sorts. He did not seem to know where he was, was drifting in and out of consciousness, and was shaking all over. Nancy tried to get Sam out of bed, but Sam couldn't move his legs very well. She had never seen him like this before. Worried, she called 911. The ambulance arrived within a few minutes, and they were off to the emergency room. After a series of laboratory and clinical tests, Sam was diagnosed with West Nile viral encephalitis.

You have just read about the basic workings of the immune system, how it tries to fight viral infections, and what kinds of processes, such as inflammation, can facilitate the entry of a virus into the nervous system. Scientists have shown that in animals infected with West Nile virus, blocking immune and inflammatory processes greatly reduces the ability of the virus to enter the nervous system, thus decreasing the development of encephalitis. This has also been shown to be true for other viruses that cause encephalitis. But what happens when a virus manages to overcome the immune system and gain entry into the nervous system? What often results are the symptoms of encephalitis.

SYMPTOMS

Symptoms of viral encephalitis often begin suddenly, a few days to a few weeks after exposure to a virus (for example, West Nile) or after reactivation of a latent viral infection (such as herpes simplex). The most common symptoms of viral encephalitis are abnormal temperature (either very high or very low), severe headaches, stiff neck, and nausea. Patients can experience changes in their mental status such as confusion and delirium, which are often among the earliest noticeable signs of encephalitis. These symptoms can eventually deteriorate into seizures, abnormal movements or tremors, lethargy, and coma. Since encephalitis can be caused by a number of different viruses and other pathogens, there are currently no accurate fatality statistics on encephalitis. However, to show just how serious encephalitis is, we can look at the fact that there is a 70% fatality rate for untreated cases of herpes virus encephalitis. Recovery from viral encephalitis can take about a month, although some patients have long-lasting neurological damage. As you read in Chapter 1, the first outbreak of West Nile virus (WNV) in North America was discovered after a small group of patients in the New York City area came down with similar symptoms of fever, changes in mental status (such as confusion and delirium), and profound muscle weakness— all characteristics of viral encephalitis.

To understand how different symptoms of encephalitis arise and are diagnosed, you need to know some basic concepts of nervous system function. The nervous system can be divided into two main anatomical parts: the **central nervous system** (CNS) and the peripheral nervous system (PNS) (Figure 4.1). The central nervous system consists of the brain and spinal cord. The peripheral nervous system is made up of a network of nerves that extends throughout the body—all the nerve cells outside of the brain and spinal cord. Together, the CNS and PNS acquire and process information from the environment,

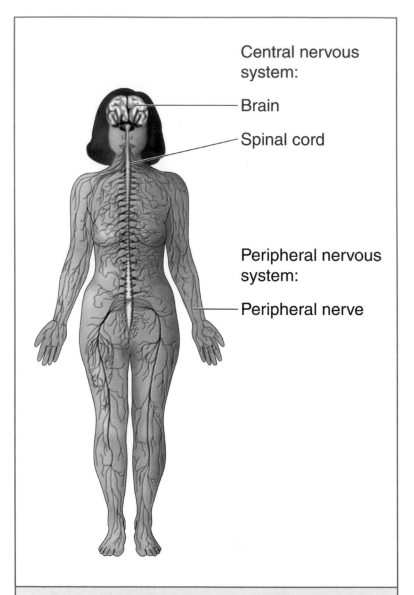

Central nervous system:

Brain

Spinal cord

Peripheral nervous system:

Peripheral nerve

Figure 4.1 The major divisions of the nervous system. The nervous system is divided into the central nervous system (CNS), which consists of the brain and spinal cord and the peripheral nervous system (PNS), which includes all of the nerves in the rest of the body.

plan how the body will react to this information, and then carry out the appropriate responses.

THE CENTRAL NERVOUS SYSTEM

The two major cell types in the CNS are nerve cells, called **neurons** and a variety of cell types that support them, collectively called **neuroglia**, or **glia** for short.

Neurons are nondividing cells that consist of a **cell body** and two types of branches called **axons** and dendrites (Figure 4.3). The cell body is the "brain" of the neuron, integrating information about what is going on around it. How does the cell body know what is going on around it? In the simplest terms, axons relay signals from the cell body to other cells and dendrites receive information from other neurons. Most neurons have only one axon and many dendrites, by which they are each connected to many other neurons. The place where neurons connect with each other and exchange information is called a **synapse** (from the Greek words *syn*, meaning "together," and *haptein*, meaning "to clasp" or "to hold"). In order to communicate with each other, neurons release signaling chemicals called neurotransmitters into the synapse, which bind to specific receptors on the surface of the neuron on the opposite side of the synapse. Each of the 100 billion neurons in the human nervous system forms 100 to 1,000 connections with other neurons. Therefore, the brain has between 10 trillion and 100 trillion synapses. Although it was once thought that synaptic connections in adult brains were relatively fixed, scientists now realize that even in adults, synapses can change and develop with use and activity. So the well-known saying that applies to muscles, "Use it or lose it," can also apply to synapses!

The brain has historically been referred to as an "immune privileged site." That means that the fluid around the cells (**extracellular fluid**) does not circulate through the normal lymphatic vessels and are not sampled in the way that fluid

(continued on page 56)

GLIA: MORE THAN JUST A SUPPORTING ROLE

When you are born, your brain already has almost all of the neurons that it will ever have and weighs approximately 400 grams (0.88 pounds). As you get older, your brain continues to grow. By the time you're an adult, your brain will weigh 1300–1400 grams (2.8–3.0 pounds)—three times what it weighed when you were born! Since neurons do not divide, how does the brain grow? The answer to this mystery is that glial cells continue to divide and grow throughout your life. This results in an increase in the overall size of the brain.

Famous scientist Albert Einstein's brain had almost twice the normal number of glial cells. So what are these cells doing? Taking their name from the Greek word for "glue," glia provide structural support and nutrients to neurons. Glia cannot produce the electrical signals, called action potentials, that neurons use to communicate. Instead, to communicate with other glia and with neurons, glial cells must release and detect chemical signals.

Scientists used to believe that glia played only a supportive role in the brain, helping neurons do the business of the nervous system. More recent studies indicate, however, that glia perform more tasks than were previously realized.

The three main types of glia in the nervous system are called astrocytes, oligodendrocytes, Schwann cells, and microglia. Astrocytes are the largest glial cells in the brain. Studies over the past 10 years have shown that astrocytes not only provide structure and nutrition to neurons but also influence the development and the activity of neurons.

Oligodendrocytes and Schwann cells make a fatty substance called myelin, which insulates the axon of a neuron and helps it to propagate electrical signals quickly and efficiently. There are many diseases that destroy the myelin (a process called "demyelination") in either the CNS or PNS. It is thought that demyelination results from an abnormal immune response in which the body starts to attack its own myelin. These diseases are considered autoimmune diseases. One common disease of demyelination is called multiple sclerosis (MS), which currently affects 2.5 million adults and children worldwide.

The **microglia** are the smallest glia in the nervous system. Microglia serve as the "immune system" for the nervous system. They rapidly destroy invading microbes or remove dead cells from the brain and spinal cord (Figure 4.2). After a nerve injury, trauma, stroke, or inflammation, microglia digest and clear dead neurons. In addition to getting rid of dead neurons and invading microbes, microglia also produce and secrete several chemical compounds, including cytokines. In the developing brain, microglia secrete growth factors that may help neurons extend their axons and dendrites. In the mature brain, activated microglia secrete signaling messenger molecules. These molecules travel freely in the brain and may help communication between cells. When too many of these messengers are produced, they can harm healthy cells. How microglia control the quality and quantity of signaling molecules they release is a current "hot" topic of scientific research.

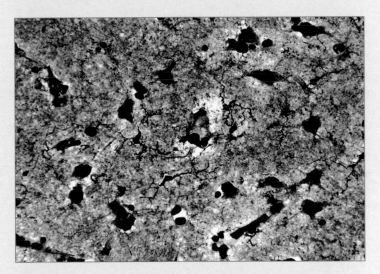

Figure 4.2 This image of a human microglial cell was taken with a light microscope (X120 magnification). Microglia, the smallest glia of the nervous system, destroy invading microbes and rapidly digest parts of dead neurons.

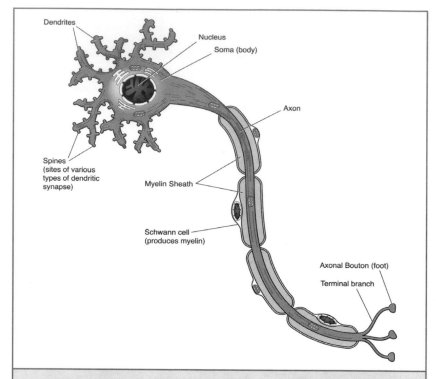

Figure 4.3 A nerve cell—also known as the neuron. The neuron consists of a cell body (called a soma) where the nucleus resides. Sprouting off of the soma there are typically several dendrites. The tips of the dendrites are called spines, which is where the neuron receives information from other neurons by making synapses. On the other side of the soma there is typically one axon, which is usually quite a bit longer than the dendrites. Axons of higher vertebrates are surrounded by a fatty substance called the myelin sheath, which provides insulation to the axon. Myelin is produced by a type of glial cell called a Schwann cell. At the end of the axon there are typically a few branches, which terminate in small bulbs called boutons, which is the place where the neuron forms synapses to send information to other neurons.

(continued from page 53)

from other organs is. However, it has been found that antigens from the brain do enter the circulation and are detected by T cells. In most cases, however, rather than reacting against them, normal brain proteins seem to instruct the cells of the immune system to tolerate brain antigens. There are some exceptions to this rule, such as in diseases like multiple sclerosis, where an inappropriate immune response is generated against a normal CNS protein called "**myelin** basic protein." The complete separation of the immune and nervous systems has also been challenged by the work of Dr. Kevin J. Tracey and his colleagues at the Northshore University Hospital in Long Island, New York over the last several years. They have shown that the immune system and the nervous system can "talk" to each other directly, exchanging signals and responding to general trends in activity in one system or the other. For example, Tracey and his colleagues have shown that activity of the vagus nerve, which helps regulate the stomach, intestines, lungs, and heart, influences the cytokine production of macrophages during an infection. Part of the mechanism by which it does this is revealed by the researchers' discovery that macrophages have neurotransmitter receptors, which were traditionally believed to exist only on neurons. This new level of communication between the immune and nervous systems has recently been dubbed "the inflammatory reflex," and is an exciting area of emerging research. Since certain viruses bind to receptors once thought to exist only on neurons, but that we now know are present on other types of cells (such as macrophages), this new area of research may also turn out to be relevant to the development of viral encephalitis.

Higher Organization of the Central Nervous System

Infection of different regions of the brain or subpopulations of neurons and glia trigger different symptoms of encephalitis. For example, tremors and movement disorders occur when neurons in areas of the brain that are known to control movement, such as the basal ganglia, are affected. Let's get a sense of the names and locations of those areas in the brain.

The nervous system is the predominant controller, regulator, and communicator of the body. The brain is the center of mental processes while the spinal cord and nerves relay information about the rest of the body to and from the brain. The nervous system can be divided into several functional systems with distinct roles: the sensory, motor, and associational systems. The **sensory systems** acquire and process information about the environment. They are the "input" systems. Sensory systems include those that process information about the five senses: sight, sound, taste, smell, and touch. The **motor systems** respond to the information taken in by the sensory systems. They are the "output" systems. Motor systems are those that control voluntary skeletal muscle movements. The **associational systems** work between the sensory and motor systems by processing the "input" information and organizing "output" responses. The three systems all work together to ensure that the body perceives the internal and external environment, and responds appropriately.

Anatomical Areas of the Central Nervous System

There are eight major areas of the CNS: the spinal cord, brain stem, cerebellum, diencephalon, cerebral cortex, basal ganglia, hippocampus, and amygdala. Starting at the bottom and working our way up, here are the names of the areas and the major functions they are thought to direct or affect. The **spinal cord** controls movement of the limbs and body as well as processes sensory information from skin, joints, and muscles. The **brain stem** is a kind of relay station between the brain and spinal cord. It controls such basic vital functions as breathing, digestion, and heart rate. It also relays movement information and is involved in many sensory and motor functions. The **cerebellum**, which sits behind the brain stem, controls many aspects of both learning and controlling movement. The **diencephalon**, which lies deep in the center of the brain, contains the thalamus and hypothalamus, which process much of the information going to the cortex, the region of the brain involving the most complex functions. The diencephalon also controls important regulatory functions like body temperature, the endocrine system, and visceral functions.

Looking at the brain from the outside, you can see two deeply folded symmetrical halves called **cerebral hemispheres**, which control many complex brain functions. The outer layer is called the **cerebral cortex** and deeper within are the **basal ganglia**, **hippocampus**, and **amygdala**. In the simplest terms, the basal ganglia regulate many aspects of movement. The hippocampus is concerned with learning and memory, and the amygdala is involved in many aspects of emotions.

Each of the cerebral hemispheres is divided into four functionally distinct lobes, which have special functions. The **frontal lobe** is involved planning and movement control, working memory, emotions, and reasoning. The **parietal lobe** processes sensory information from the environment. The **temporal lobe** is mostly involved in hearing, while the **occipital lobe** (*oculus* is the Latin word for "eye") integrates many features of visual information. There are also many more structures that lay deep inside of the brain, which process information about memories, emotions, and sleep, among other things.

Now you can see why a viral infection located in the CNS can have such complicated consequences such as the symptoms of encephalitis—which can range from cognitive impairments and sensory perception changes to personality changes and movement disorders—because the CNS has so many diverse and crucial functions (Figure 4.4).

VIRAL ENTRY INTO THE CENTRAL NERVOUS SYSTEM

As mentioned earlier, many different kinds of viruses can cause encephalitis. But encephalitis does not occur in every person infected with those viruses. The reasons for this are not completely understood. However, what is known is that to cause encephalitis, a virus first has to gain access to the central nervous system.

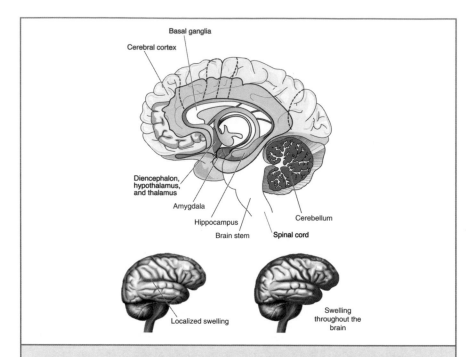

Figure 4.4 Diagram of the central nervous system. A lateral view of the brain and spinal cord showing the seven major components of the CNS. Starting at the spinal cord and working our way up, here are the names of the major regions and the functions they are thought to direct or effect. The spinal cord controls movement as well as processes sensory information from skin, joints and muscles. The brain stem relays information between the brain and spinal cord. It controls such basic vital functions as breathing, digestion, and heart rate. The cerebellum, which sits behind the brainstem, controls many aspects of both learning and controlling movement. The diencephalon contains the thalamus and hypothalamus, which process much of the information going to the cortex, the region of the brain involved in the most complex functions. The diencephalon also controls important regulatory functions like body temperature, the endocrine system, and visceral functions. From the outside, the brain displays very folded symmetrical halves called cerebral hemispheres, which control many complex brain functions. The outer layer is called the cerebral cortex and deeper within are the basal ganglia, hippocampus, and amygdala. In the simplest terms, the basal ganglia regulate many aspects of movement, the hippocampus is involved in learning and memory, and the amygdala is involved in many aspects of emotions. The location in the brain where encephalitis begins may therefore have very different effects on the patient.

In general, there are two routes that viruses can take to get into the nervous system: They can travel either through nerves themselves or via the bloodstream. A virus may exploit a seemingly innocuous injury such as an insect bite or cold sore as a route into an exposed nerve. Once inside a neuron, the virus can "hitchhike" on the normal transport pathways that neurons use to move molecules and organelles (intracellular structures that are sort of like the "body parts" of a cell) around within themselves, or a virus can spread from one neuron to another via synapses.

Some viruses, such as the rabies virus, gain entry into neurons by sticking to cellular receptors that are found on many neurons and are normally used by the cell for detecting neurotransmitters. The face, which has a high concentration of nerves, is a particularly common point of CNS entry for viruses that cause encephalitis. For example, herpes simplex virus-1 (HSV-1), which causes cold sores, can gain access to the nervous system by spreading from a cold sore around the mouth into the trigeminal nerve, which provides sensation to the mouth and other parts of the face.

As just mentioned, routes of nutrition, which exchange cells and materials with the CNS, are particularly vulnerable to viral infection. There are two systems that serve to bring nutrients and oxygen to the cells of the CNS—the blood and the cerebrospinal fluid.

The Blood-Brain Barrier (BBB)

Viruses can enter the blood directly, such as when a mosquito carrying a virus bites your arm. Once in the blood, viruses can infect different kinds of blood cells or travel freely through the plasma until they reach a cell that has the right receptor with which they can interact. Many of the cells in the blood are part of the immune system and are thus "professional soldiers" in the body's war against infection. It is only when these cellular defenses fail that a viral infection can take hold in the CNS.

(continued on page 64)

THE HUMAN IMMUNE SYSTEM

The human immune system consists of a complex set of cells and processes that help protect us against disease. There are several different aspects of the immune system.

The body's first "line of defense" against infection consists of physical barriers that prevent pathogens (such as viruses that might lead to encephalitis) from getting inside the cells. The largest barrier is the skin. Other barriers include the mucous membranes (which can trap pathogens in sticky mucus and help get them out of the body through coughing, sneezing, or urination and defecation) and cilia (hair-like structures found in the nose, lungs, and other organs that help "sweep" foreign materials out of the body). Before it can get into a cell and start an infection, a virus or other pathogen has to make it past these barriers. Frequently, a cut or open wound provides the entryway the pathogen needs to get into the bloodstream.

Once the pathogen has invaded the body, the immune system's "second line of defense" kicks in. This part of the immune system is made up of many different kinds of cells, all of which play a unique role in combating infection. Among the immune cells that attack the invader first are macrophages—large cells that literally gobble up invading organisms and kill them. Other immune cells are called lymphocytes (also known as B cells and T cells). B cells travel constantly through the blood, on the look-out for foreign substances that may have entered the body. When they find cells or particles they do not recognize (known as antigens), they attach to them and produce antibodies—the proteins that stay in the body even after the infection is over to help the immune system "remember" a certain pathogen if it ever enters the body again. Meanwhile, there are two kinds of T cells that help the second line of defense. Helper T cells find invading pathogens and send out chemical signals to let the immune system know a foreign substance is in the body. Killer T cells attach to and destroy cells they don't recognize—whether these cells are viruses, bacteria, or some other kind of pathogen.

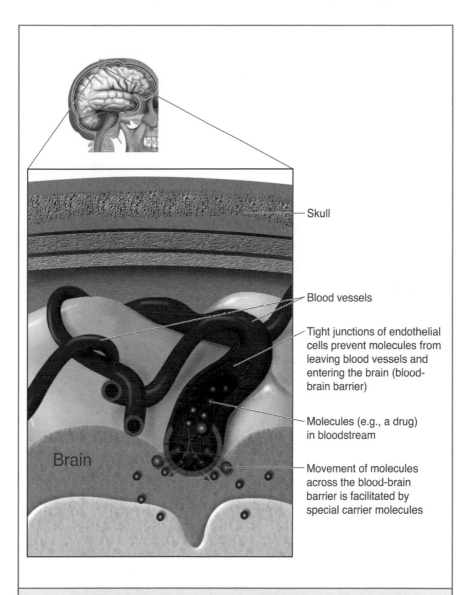

Skull

Blood vessels

Tight junctions of endothelial cells prevent molecules from leaving blood vessels and entering the brain (blood-brain barrier)

Molecules (e.g., a drug) in bloodstream

Movement of molecules across the blood-brain barrier is facilitated by special carrier molecules

Brain

Figure 4.5 The blood-brain barrier. The blood-brain barrier is formed by cells called endothelial cells that line the blood vessels in the brain. These cells form tight junctions through which only very small molecules, such as nutrients, can pass. The blood-brain barrier is very important in keeping viruses and other pathogens from entering the brain and causing encephalitis.

(continued from page 61)

There is one anatomical structure in the brain that is particularly relevant to viral encephalitis: the blood-brain barrier (BBB) (Figure 4.5). The BBB is a network of blood vessels that create a membrane that serves as a boundary between the cells of the brain and the bloodstream that flows throughout the rest of the body. The BBB lets some kinds of substances (like oxygen) into the brain, but keeps other substances (like some harmful drugs or microorganisms) out. Scientists have shown that many viruses enter the brain by crossing the BBB. Traffic of immune cells across the BBB to survey the area is tightly regulated under normal conditions, but during a viral infection it is thought that a "Trojan horse" strategy can allow viruses to cross the BBB. In other words, cells from the blood infected with a virus, such as West Nile Virus (WNV) or HIV, move through the BBB, exposing neurons and glia in the CNS to the virus. The general process of inflammation then ensues. In the brain itself, the resident white blood cells (**microglia**) and brain macrophages can produce cytokines that can help cause inflammation. These cells are themselves susceptible to infection by viruses and can encounter infected cells that have entered the brain from the blood. As in other tissues, the inflammatory reaction triggered by a localized viral infection can cause the blood vessels that make up the BBB to leak, allowing more virus particles into the CNS. Other, smaller blood vessels that contact the CNS can serve as routes of entry into the brain when they are functioning irregularly due to inflammation.

THE CHOROID PLEXUS AND CEREBROSPINAL FLUID

Cerebrospinal fluid (**CSF**) bathes the brain and spinal cord, functioning as a shock-absorbing cushion against the skull as well as providing nutrients to the brain and spinal cord. This fluid maintains the extracellular environment for neurons and glia and may also function as a kind of local lymphatic system. In a normal healthy individual, there is a blood-CSF barrier maintained by the epithelium in the **choroid plexus**, an area within each brain ventricle that produces most of the CSF. It has been found that viruses can also enter the CNS through the choroid plexus.

In this chapter, you have learned about the cells that make up the CNS and how the major structures of the brain are organized. You have also learned how viruses can gain entry into the nervous system, such as by infecting neurons directly or by entering the CNS through the bloodstream, CSF, or across the blood-brain barrier. Now that you know the different regions of the brain and what kinds of higher functions they control, you can easily imagine how the symptoms of encephalitis occur and why they can be either relatively mild or very serious, depending on which part of the brain is infected. In the next chapter, you will learn how doctors diagnose and treat encephalitis.

5

Diagnosis and Treatment of Encephalitis

You now know how the immune system attempts to fight off viruses and how viruses get into the nervous system. But what happens once they get there? Inflammation in the brain leads to many molecular, cellular, and clinical changes in a person who is suffering from encephalitis. So how do doctors detect these changes and diagnose encephalitis? What can they do to help the patient?

DIAGNOSIS

For any known infectious disease, the Centers for Disease Control and Prevention (CDC) establishes guidelines for its detection, treatment, and surveillance. Therefore, a health-care provider has a framework with which to approach a patient suspected of having viral encephalitis (or any other disease). The first recommended approach for diagnosing a person with the symptoms of viral encephalitis is to try to rule out another possible cause for the condition. For example, a person who has had a stroke might experience symptoms similar to those of encephalitis. Although the criteria used to identify the various viruses that cause encephalitis may differ, the general principles are the same. For our purposes, we will examine how a diagnosis of West Nile virus encephalitis is made.

White Blood Cell Count

Someone suspected of having West Nile virus infection generally has a higher than normal white blood cell count in the CSF, a condition referred to as **pleocytosis**; an altered mental state that lasts more than a day; and signs of CNS inflammation, including a very high or very low temperature. Neuroimaging tests will show acute inflammation of the brain and spinal cord or **demyelination**, seizures, or other abnormal symptoms.

The CDC criteria has outlined specific criteria for arboviral encephalitis which is the kind of encephalitis caused by the West Nile Virus (see the Box on page 68), which health professionals should consult as part of their process of diagnosis. In addition to these symptoms, several laboratory tests, described in the next sections, must be performed to confirm the diagnosis.

Medical History

With any suspected infectious disease, a good medical professional begins by gathering extensive epidemiological information from the patient. *Epidemiology* refers to the study of the incidence and distribution of disease. The health-care provider conducts an interview with the patient to establish the patient's "history." (If the patient is physically unable to respond to questions, a close family member is usually interviewed.) The health care provider asks what kinds of illnesses the patient has had during his or her life, discusses the person's vaccination record, family history, and whether the person has any underlying physical conditions, such as diabetes, that might put him or her at risk for certain kinds of diseases. Telling the physician about recent travels or outdoor activities is important, because the patient may have been exposed to a new infectious organism during these experiences. Even the season during which illness begins can be an important clue in the diagnosis, since different pathogens thrive under different environmental conditions. As you'll remember from Chapter 1, the first patients with West Nile virus in North America during the summer of 1999 all lived near each other and had recently spent time outdoors in areas with lots of mosquitoes that were later found to have harbored the West Nile virus.

Clinical Examination and Tests

Once the patient's history is taken, a series of clinical examinations is performed. In cases where viral encephalitis is suspected, the health-care provider should conduct a physical examination of the patient, looking for cuts, scrapes, bites, or other physical signs of sites at which a pathogen such as a virus might have gained access to the nervous system.

CDC CRITERIA FOR DIAGNOSING ARBOVIRAL ENCEPHALITIS

CLINICAL DESCRIPTION

Arboviral infections may be asymptomatic [showing no symptoms] or may result in illnesses of varying severity sometimes associated with the central nervous system (CNS). When the CNS is affected, clinical syndromes ranging from fever and headache to meningitis to encephalitis may occur, and these are usually indistinguishable from similar syndromes caused by other viruses. (As you remember, meningitis is an inflammation of the tissue around the brain and spinal cord.) Arboviral meningitis is characterized by fever, headache, stiff neck, and pleocytosis. Arboviral encephalitis is characterized by fever, headache, and altered mental states, ranging from confusion to coma (e.g., partial or full paralysis, cranial nerve palsies, sensory deficits, abnormal reflexes, generalized convulsions, and abnormal movements).

LABORATORY CRITERIA FOR DIAGNOSIS

- Fourfold or greater change in virus-specific counts antibody within the blood, or

Different tests provide measurements of the general level of dysfunction and areas of the nervous system that are affected. You have probably had some of these tests yourself during a routine physical. For example, standard tests are performed to assess hearing and vision, reflexes (hitting the knee with a small rubber hammer), balance, motor coordination, mental status, and behavior. For a patient suspected of

- Isolation of virus from or demonstration of specific viral antigen or viral DNA sequences in tissue, blood, cerebrospinal fluid (CSF), or other body fluid, or

- Virus-specific immunoglobulin M (IgM) antibodies demonstrated in CSF, or

- Virus-specific IgM antibodies demonstrated in serum and confirmed by demonstration of virus-specific serum immunoglobulin G (IgG) antibodies in the same or a later specimen.

CASE CLASSIFICATION

Probable: an encephalitis or meningitis case occurring during a period when arboviral transmission is likely, and with the following supportive blood work: 1) a single or stable (less than or equal to twofold change) but elevated concentration of virus-specific serum antibodies; or 2) serum IgM antibodies detected by one method but not yet by another diagnostic procedure.

Confirmed: an encephalitis or meningitis case that is laboratory confirmed

Adapted from: Centers for Disease Control and Prevention, Division of Public Health Surveillance and Informatics. Available online at *http://www.cdc.gov/epo/dphsi/casedef/encephalitiscurrent.htm*.

having viral encephalitis, an electroencephalogram (EEG) is recommended, which measures the electrical activity of the brain. For a routine EEG, 20 pairs of electrodes are placed all over the patient's scalp at certain positions to register the activity of different brain regions (Figure 5.1). The test records the amount of voltage between each pair of electrodes, giving an indication of how much neural activity is taking place in different brain regions. In patients with encephalitis, an EEG is often abnormal, showing differences in brain activity in various areas, depending on which part of the CNS is affected. For example, some patients with encephalitis experience seizures. During a seizure, an EEG would show more electrical activity in the brain than normal.

In addition to testing electrical activity, neurologists have several different non-invasive ways of imaging the brain to help assess physical abnormalities such as brain inflammation or hemorrhaging. A computerized axial tomography (CAT) scan uses focused X rays, detectors, and computers to collect a series of two-dimensional images through the brain. This method can give a general picture of many brain structures at the resolution of millimeters. The images generated by a CAT scan can give evidence of viral encephalitis as well as other causes of similar neurological symptoms, such as brain tumors, seizures, or stroke (Figure 5.2).

Another standard tool of neurological evaluation is called magnetic resonance imaging, or MRI. An MRI generates images by applying magnetic fields to the brain, causing hydrogen molecules to align in characteristic ways. Changes from the normal patterns of alignment can also help localize the regions of inflammation in the nervous system. Different viruses that cause encephalitis are known to produce characteristic kinds of changes in an MRI.

In addition to looking at the brain, other organ systems must also be examined in order to rule out nonviral causes of encephalitis. For example, a chest X ray is routinely taken

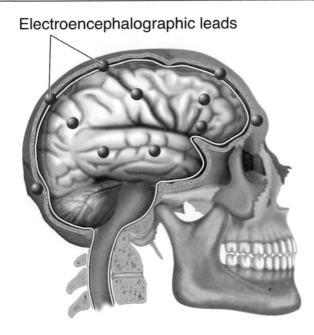

Electroencephalographic leads

Figure 5.1 Neurologists' Toolbox: Electroencephalogram (EEG). The electroencephalogram (EEG) represents the voltage recorded between two electrodes applied to the scalp. Typically, 19 pairs of electrodes (electroencephalographic leads) are placed at standard positions distributed all over the head. The recording obtained from each pair of electrodes is a bit different because each electrode samples the activity of a population of neurons in a different brain region. In patients with viral encephalitis, the inflammation of the brain will lead to changes in the normal electrical activity of the brain. These changes can be measured through an EEG.

and, if it is abnormal, then other causes of encephalitis—such as infection by bacteria, rickettsia (ticks or lice), fungi, or other parasites which might cause lung inflammation—are investigated.

Cellular and Molecular Diagnosis

Different viruses tend to favor specific tissues or cell types in the body so different organs may need to be tested to

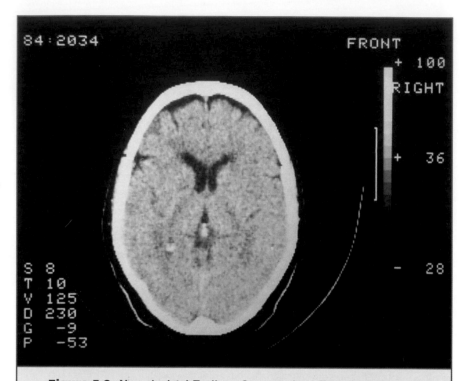

Figure 5.2 Neurologists' Toolbox: Computerized Tomography (CT scan). In computerized tomography, the X-ray source and detectors are moved around the patient's head. This type of X-ray scan generates a grid of intersecting points that have been obtained from several directions. The signal at each point can then be computed, allowing reconstruction of a "slice" through the brain that preserves three-dimensional relationships. This CT scan shows a section of a normal adult brain.

determine the type of virus causing a case of encephalitis. For example, arboviruses like West Nile virus live in the blood and elicit certain kinds of antibodies that can be found in the **sera** (the fluid part of the blood). Herpes simplex viruses may be found in the brain itself, so a brain **biopsy** (removing a small piece of tissue and analyzing it) or other molecular tests are necessary. Blood, urine, and other body fluids may be sampled to try to detect a foreign organism.

For example, both cerebrospinal fluid and serum are extracted from the patient and examined in a laboratory. The CSF is tested for the presence of bacteria or blood cells. Then the numbers and types of white blood cells present are counted. Usually, a person with an infection in the CNS will have a high number of cells in his or her CSF. If this is the case, then the types of white blood cells present are often determined using antibodies to signature molecules on their surface. This procedure is referred to as flow cytometry. Knowing what kind of white blood cells are present in the CSF and their ratio can give clues to the type or stage of infection. Like the CSF, the blood is tested for elevated numbers of white blood cells, a condition called "leukocytosis." Blood sugar levels are also measured because low levels can indicate that a bacterial or fungal infection is taking place.

MOLECULAR DIAGNOSIS
Polymerase Chain Reaction
Basic biological studies often lead to dramatic improvements in medical care. As mentioned in Chapter 2, the genomes of many infectious organisms, such as bacteria and viruses, are now known. This knowledge, coupled with other advances in molecular biology, has led to improvements in the way diseases such as viral infections are diagnosed. Pieces of viral genomes (their nucleic acids) can now be detected from blood, CSF, and body tissues. In 1988, Nobel laureate Kary Mullis invented a technique called the polymerase chain reaction (PCR), which makes it possible to amplify known sequences of genes from nucleic acids isolated from cells. PCR works by repeatedly copying a small stretch of DNA, using each amplified bit of DNA as a template for another round of duplication. With this method, a billion copies of the same section of DNA can be collected in a test tube in a matter of hours (Figure 5.3). The original DNA template can be isolated from human cells or from any other organism. Because it is indeed a molecular "chain reaction," the technique allows even very low levels of

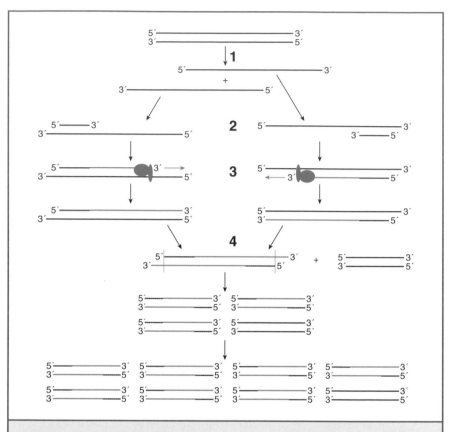

Figure 5.3 Polymerase Chain Reaction (PCR) helps to identify the viral cause of encephalitis. PCR is a technique used to copy a tiny piece of DNA in a test tube many million times. DNA strands have a beginning and an end, referred to as 5' and 3'. The mirror image strand is always paired with the first strand. The cycle of replication has three steps: (1) The DNA sample is heated, which makes the DNA strands fall apart so that they can be read off again and copied. (2) To do this, two short pieces of DNA called oligonucleotides are made so that they stick to opposite strands of the DNA piece that is being replicated. (3) At the points of contact an added enzyme called DNA polymerase can start to read off the genetic code and link code words through which two new double strands of DNA are formed. (4) The procedure is then repeated many times, doubling at each step the number of copies of the desired DNA segment. PCR makes it possible to discover very small amounts of viral DNA in a human cell, so that it is possible to diagnose the presence of a particular virus in a patient within hours of obtaining a sample.

viral nucleic acids to be detected, making it an increasingly useful tool in clinical diagnostic laboratories.

ELISA

The most accepted molecular method used to help diagnose viral encephalitis is called an IgM capture enzyme-linked immunosorbent assay (ELISA). It sounds complicated, but an ELISA is really just a way of detecting the antibodies that your body makes as part of the normal immune response. As you know, an antibody is a protein made by a type of white blood cell called a B cell. These proteins, called immunoglobulins (Ig), are made when a B cell encounters firsthand or learns from another cell that a foreign molecule (antigen) or pathogen is present. The antibody specifically binds to the foreign molecule or organism, killing it or flagging it for other cells in the immune system to detect and kill. Throughout the course of an infection, different types of antibodies are made. The first type secreted into the blood by B cells during an infection is called immunoglobulin M (IgM). By detecting the amount of specific IgM in a patient's blood, medical professionals can tell if the patient is suffering an acute infection. In the case of West Nile virus, most infected patients will have detectable amounts of IgM against the virus in their blood after about eight days of infection. These antibodies can last for one to two months, and sometimes longer. Within three weeks, another type of antibody, called IgG, will be present in the blood of most infected patients. This kind of antibody can also be detected in samples from the patient.

Taken together, all of these tests, from the clinical history, to the brain imaging techniques, to cultures from blood, CSF, and molecular diagnostic tests like PCR and ELISA, help a doctor diagnose encephalitis.

TREATMENT

Treatment for viral encephalitis is largely nonspecific and "supportive," which means that it tries to favor the overall health of the patient rather than specifically targeting the virus itself. This is because viruses hide out in cells, so most medications that will attack the virus will also harm the patient's own cells. Pain medication is often prescribed, as are drugs—such as corticosteroids and carbohydrates (mannitol)—that help control inflammation and swelling. Antiseizure medications (also called anticonvulsants) may also be prescribed. Patients

AWAKENINGS

For a very poignant portrayal of patients with encephalitis, and a medical doctor's struggle to help them, watch the movie *Awakenings*. Based on a book by Dr. Oliver Sacks, a neurologist and writer, this movie stars Robert DeNiro as a patient and Robin Williams as Dr. Sacks. When the neurologist first arrives at his new clinical assignment, some of these patients have not moved for years! The reasons for this were not clear. After carefully reading the patients' charts, Sacks noticed that all of these paralyzed patients in this nursing home facility had suffered from childhood viral encephalitis during the influenza epidemic of 1918. He investigated other reports of such patients and contacted their physicians to compare notes. He came to believe there is a connection between viral infection and the body's mechanisms for controlling movement. Through his investigations, Sacks learned of a newly discovered neurotransmitter (the kind of chemical that neurons use to communicate) called dopamine. Dopamine is released by certain nerve cells involved in generating movement. The lack of movement or uncoordinated movements of Sack's patients suggested that their brains were depleted of dopamine. Sacks treated his paralyzed patients with experimental doses of a chemical compound called levodopa (L-DOPA), which gets modified by proteins in the brain to become dopamine. (The person who may also need to be supported with intravenous fluids and respiratory aid (a ventilator).

There are a few specific antiviral medications that are also available. If the influenza virus is to blame, then a drug called amantadine is given. This drug works only against influenza virus—not any other viruses. It inhibits a viral protein called the M2 protein, which forms a channel in the virus membrane.

discovered dopamine, as well as the drug L-DOPA, was a Swedish doctor named Arvid Carlsson. Carlsson shared the Nobel Prize for these discoveries in the year 2000.) Temporarily, and with varying degrees of success, Sacks was able to restore some higher functions to many of the patients. Some of the patients were able to tolerate this drug for long periods of time, while others were not. Regardless of the individual success of the patients, the overall study helped to establish L-DOPA as a treatment for patients with Parkinson's disease (a condition in which the neurons that make dopamine are lost or damaged) or similar symptoms. This treatment or derivatives of it are still in use today.

There is still an open question about the connection between previous viral infections and the development of Parkinson's disease or Parkinson's-like symptoms. For example, the TV and movie star Michael J. Fox developed Parkinson's disease at a very young age, along with three of his childhood coworkers. The chance that four relatively young people would come down with Parkinson's seems to be an unlikely coincidence and fuels the hypothesis that perhaps they shared an underlying viral infection during their childhood. It is also well known that people who have suffered from Japanese encephalitis and other arboviruses such as West Nile virus, may develop Parkinson's-like symptoms.

The influenza (flu) virus needs this protein to replicate once it gets inside a cell, so amantadine slows viral replication. If encephalitis is caused by herpes simplex virus infection, an antiviral drug called acyclovir is prescribed. Acyclovir is a compound that is related to, but not identical to, a viral DNA nucleotide. Therefore, its incorporation into the viral DNA stops it replication. In this way, acyclovir specifically targets virally-infected cells. Although the use of this drug has radically improved the outcome of HSV-induced encephalitis, there is still a high mortality (death) rate (around 28%). Most patients recover from encephalitis within a month or so. Though most cases of encephalitis can be treated successfully, there are still some major health risks associated with viral encephalitis. For example, up to 35% of people who contract encephalitis from the eastern equine encephalitis virus will die.

6

Viral Encephalitis

INTRODUCTION

According to the World Health Organization (WHO), there are at least 50,000 serious cases of viral encephalitis annually in Asia alone, of which 10,000 are fatal. Although different viruses are more prevalent than others in various parts of the world, the general symptoms of encephalitis are always similar. In this chapter, we will review some of the different kinds of viruses that can cause encephalitis. As examples, the viruses that cause most cases of encephalitis in the United States are examined in more detail. These viruses are enteroviruses, herpes simplex viruses, rabies virus, and the arboviruses, of which the most relevant is West Nile virus.

VIRAL CAUSES

Enteroviruses

Enteroviruses, which include the **poliovirus, Coxsackie virus,** and **echoviruses,** establish infection within the gastrointestinal (GI) tract. The gastrointestinal tract is also called the "enteric" tract, which gives this family of viruses their name. Enteroviruses have genomes made of RNA, like many of the other viruses that can cause encephalitis. The genomes enter the host cell, get copied, and are then turned into proteins that are needed to make more RNA.

Poliovirus

Poliovirus belongs to a subgroup of enteroviruses called *Picornaviridae*. (*Pico* means "small" in Latin, and *RNA* stands for the form of viral genome.) There are three types of poliovirus. All of them can spread from the gut via the lymphatics to the blood and then to the CNS. In the CNS, poliovirus infects motor neurons of the spinal cord and brain stem, resulting in inflammation, the death of neurons, and subsequent loss of movement. The time between the start of the infection and the development of symptoms ranges from 3 to 35 days. The severity of the symptoms also varies widely. Most infections are **asymptomatic** (showing no symptoms). Even without symptoms, infected people can transmit the virus, which is excreted in their feces. Those patients who do experience paralysis can often recover significant function with physical therapy, because surviving neurons grow new connections to restore muscle function.

The first cases of polio were described at the end of the 18th century in Great Britain, and the first major outbreak in the United States was recorded in 1843, although paralytic infectious diseases—which may have been caused by polioviruses—have been recorded for thousands of years. In 1916, poliovirus was the cause of paralysis in 27,000 Americans, and claimed the lives of 6,000 more. In the 1950s, at least 20,000 Americans were suffering from polio each year. Since a vaccine was developed and administered to prevent the disease in the mid-1950s, the number of polio victims has dropped dramatically. Until recently, fewer than 500 people were infected with polio worldwide making it a rare cause of viral encephalitis. However, disruption of immunization programs in Africa from 2001 to 2004 led to a rapid increase in that number, which prompted international health organizations to initiate aggressive vaccination campaigns in 2004.

Herpes Simplex Viruses

The ancient Greeks used the word *herpes,* meaning to "creep" or "crawl," to describe the way the sores caused by these viruses appear around the lips or genitals. There are more than 100 known members of the *Herpesviridae* family. All of the viruses have large DNA genomes, and they all infect vertebrates. Several members of the herpes simplex virus family cause common diseases, including herpes simplex 1 and 2 (cold sores and genital herpes, respectively), varicella zoster (chicken pox and shingles), cytomegalovirus, and Epstein-Barr virus (mononucleosis). Each of these viruses kills the cells it infects through lysis (bursting), which is what leads to the outbreak of sores. In different cells, herpes viruses can enter a latent phase (as described in Chapter 2), sometimes for decades, and can remain in the body undetected and without producing any symptoms. It is important to note, however, that the viruses may sometimes still be spread from person to person, even if no symptoms are present. When the infection reactivates, these viruses can infect neurons and cause encephalitis. Most cases of encephalitis in the United States are caused by herpes simplex virus 1 or 2, described here in more detail.

Herpes simplex 1 (HSV-1) infects 50–90% of all adults in the entire world. It is the cause of the common cold sore, can be spread from person to person, and is the most frequent cause of viral encephalitis in developed countries. HSV-1 and the closely related HSV-2 are responsible for about 2,000 cases of encephalitis each year in the United States, with most of the cases being caused when a latent infection becomes reactivated. In the case of HSV-1, the virus can travel into the CNS through sensory nerves in the face (the trigeminal nerve) or nose (**olfactory neurons**). When a latent infection gets reactivated, the virus then travels down the nerve cell and infects non-neuronal cells around that neuron. The areas of the brain most affected are the frontal and temporal lobes above the ears, which means that hearing and movement may be affected. Symptoms include headache, fever, seizures, partial paralysis, and altered consciousness. Although this virus is the most common cause of encephalitis in the Western world, it is also the only one for which a specific medication is available. As you have already read, the drug used to treat HSV

(continued on page 84)

POLIO VICTIM BECOMES PRESIDENT OF THE UNITED STATES

In the summer of 1921, when Franklin D. Roosevelt (FDR) was 39 years old, he enjoyed a day of sailing and swimming with his family. When he got home, he felt somewhat more tired than usual and went to bed early. By the next morning, he had a fever of 102°F and could not move his legs. It soon became clear that FDR had contracted poliomyelitis, a disease named for its damage to motor neurons in the spinal cord (in Greek, *polio* means "gray" and *myelo* means "spinal cord;" motor neurons in the spinal cord are gray in color). This infection left FDR paralyzed from the waist down for the rest of his life (Figure 6.1).

Determined to walk again, FDR undertook a strict regimen of physical therapy at a resort in Georgia. He eventually bought the resort and set it up as a rehabilitation center for polio victims, where many successfully used physical therapy to strengthen the connections between their muscles and surviving motor neurons. After dedicating seven years to this center, FDR reentered public life and successfully ran for governor of New York State, where he served from 1928 to 1932. In 1932, FDR was elected president of the United States, an office he held for 12 years—longer than anyone before or since. Interestingly, because there was no television at the time, few Americans realized that FDR was paralyzed, since they rarely, if ever, saw him in person, and because he took pains to avoid being photographed in his wheelchair.

Throughout his tenure as president, FDR promoted legislation to provide services to promote the rights of the disabled. In 1934, a friend of the president, named Basil O'Connor, started a campaign to raise money for polio research. His efforts eventually culminated in the establishment of the National Foundation for Infantile Paralysis, later known as the March of Dimes. Money that American citizens donated to the organization helped fund the research that led to the development of vaccines against the polio virus, developed in the late 1950s and the early 1960s, first by Dr. Jonas Salk and then by Dr. Albert Sabin. The March of Dimes still exists. In 2001, it raised more than $26 million for scientific research.

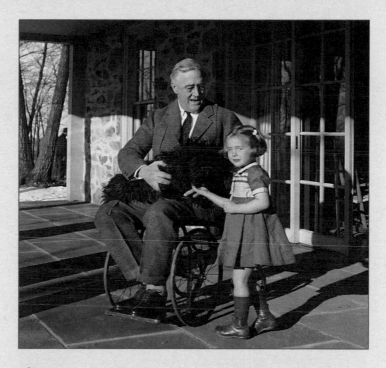

Figure 6.1 Franklin Delano Roosevelt, (FDR), paralyzed for most of his adult life after infection by the polio virus, served as president of the United States. FDR was aware of a common prejudice at that time: that people suffering from paralysis were weaker human beings. To avoid dealing with this unfounded prejudice, he usually did not allow photographs like this one to be taken, showing him in his wheelchair. As FDR proved by being the longest serving President in U.S. history, and as many others confined to a wheelchair have also shown, real strength cannot be measured by physical abilities.

(continued from page 81)

is called acyclovir. It works by slowing the multiplication of viral DNA. Acyclovir must be taken within the first 48 hours after symptoms appear. If left untreated, encephalitis from HSV has a 50–75% mortality rate and almost all survivors experience long-term neurological defects that range from mild symptoms to paralysis (Figure 6.2).

Rabies Virus

Cases of rabies have been documented throughout the world since the 23rd century B.C. The rabies virus is a member of the *genus Lyssavirus* and is fatal to humans and animals. Worldwide, more than 50,000 people die of rabies each year and 1 million people are exposed.

Rabies virus is harbored in the saliva of an infected animal and transmitted to a human by its bite. The animals that most commonly carry rabies include dogs, raccoons, skunks, and possibly bats. Infection is established at the place where the person was bitten. The location of the infection is crucial to the course of the disease, and it is the infection of motor neuron populations that can lead to paralysis. Rabies virus specifically interacts with a neurotransmitter receptor that is very common on many neurons, whereby it gains access to the neuron. The rabies virus can then spread to different parts of the CNS, causing encephalitis. If left untreated, bites to the face and head result in the majority of all rabies cases. The time from infection to the development of symptoms can vary widely, from a few days to years. Indeed, only recently have medical experts discovered that rabies virus can establish a latent infection. Once in the CNS, the disease can be spread to many other organs. In developed countries, domesticated dogs are vaccinated to prevent them from getting rabies and being able to spread it to humans. Due to a lag time between exposure and the onset of symptoms, vaccination to humans is given after exposure, together with antirabies antibodies.

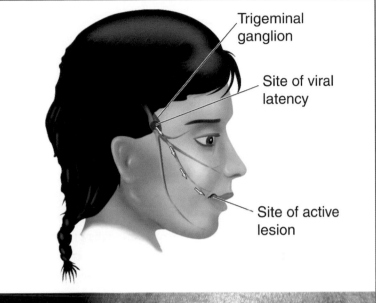

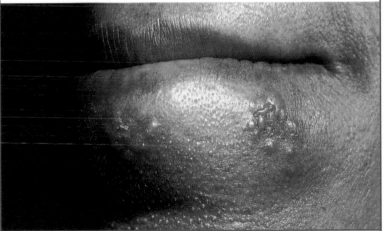

Figure 6.2 The herpes simplex virus, the virus that causes cold sores, "hides out" between outbreaks in nerves of the body called the trigeminal ganglion. Although most people infected with this virus will suffer only from bouts of painful cold sores (as pictured in the bottom photo) when the virus becomes stimulated, some people experience much more serious complications when the herpes virus spreads from the trigeminal nerve to the brain. In such cases, the result can be encephalitis.

Arboviruses
What Are Arboviruses?

The term **arbovirus** refers to an arthropod-borne virus. Arboviruses are usually spread by blood-sucking insects—such as mosquitoes or ticks. Because the term *arbovirus* refers to how the disease is spread rather than the viruses' scientific characteristics, arboviruses can belong to different virus families. Three arbovirus families can cause encephalitis in humans: *Togaviridae*, *Flaviviridae*, and *Bunyaviridae*.

Arboviruses have a complicated **zoonotic** life cycle, meaning they are spread between animals and people (Figure 6.3). The insects that transmit them are referred to as "**vectors**." The viruses in question don't cause any signs of illness in the vectors, so the vectors often serve as safe havens for viral replication. Because the vectors themselves frequently have a seasonal life cycle, arboviruses are often most commonly spread when the vector is most prevalent. For example, in the United States, viruses carried by mosquitoes are most prevalent during the summer months, when mosquitoes are breeding and the mosquito population is at its highest.

In the winter, or during whichever season their vector is least present, some arboviruses infect other intermediate hosts, such as birds or pigs, which are referred to as "**reservoirs**." The virus can then be transmitted back to a mosquito and then to a human or other animal when the mosquito feeds on the person or animal's blood. Infected people usually do not have high enough amounts of circulating virus (**viremia**) to be contagious to other people.

Epidemiology of Arboviruses

Arboviruses are present worldwide. Although only a minority (10%) of people infected by an arbovirus develops encephalitis, the absolute numbers are quite high, because of the viruses' contagious nature and widespread geographical distribution. The most deadly member of this group is the Japanese

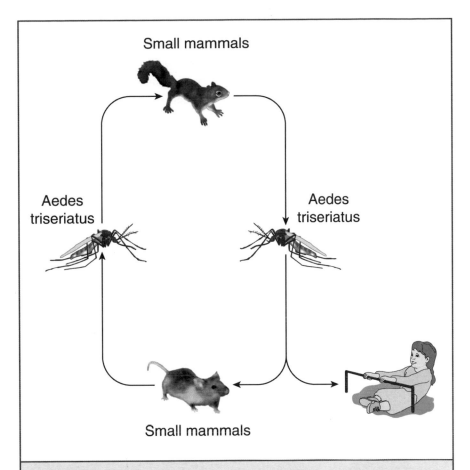

Small mammals

Aedes
triseriatus

Aedes
triseriatus

Small mammals

Figure 6.3 Zoonotic Life Cycle of an arbovirus. Arthropod-borne viruses, or arboviruses, are viruses that are maintained in nature through biological transmission between susceptible vertebrate hosts (e.g., humans) by blood feeding arthropods such as mosquitoes. Vertebrate infection occurs when the infected arthropod takes a blood meal. All arboviruses are maintained in complex life cycles involving a nonhuman vertebrate host such as a squirrel, bird or mouse, and a primary arthropod vector like a mosquito. Mosquitoes are arboviral carriers (vectors) that become infected when they feed on infected small mammals (reservoirs). Infected mosquitoes can then spread arbovirus to humans when they bite them and other animals when they bite. Humans and domestic animals can develop illnesses, including encephalitis, but usually are "dead-end" hosts because they do not produce significant viremia, and do not contribute to the transmission cycle.

MOLECULAR MIMICRY

Imitation has been called the most sincere form of flattery. It is also a successful strategy for survival. Many viruses make the same or similar versions of molecules as the cells they are infecting, in a process referred to as **"molecular mimicry."** This ability to produce materials that look identical to their host cell at the molecular level can trick the host into recognizing particles made by the virus as something that belongs to the host. This can either help the virus hide from the immune system or set off an inappropriate immune response. Viral infections are suspected or known to trigger some auto-immune diseases—conditions in which the body mistakenly attacks its own cells as it would attack a foreign pathogen.

encephalitis virus, which causes 30,000–50,000 cases of encephalitis each year in Asia, resulting in 10,000 deaths. Other medically relevant arboviruses are the equine encephalitis viruses (eastern, western, and Venezuelan), the La Crosse encephalitis virus, the St. Louis encephalitis virus (found in North and South America), the Murray Valley virus (Australia and New Zealand), and the West Nile virus (North America, Europe, Middle East, and Africa).

7

Prevention of Encephalitis

As you read in Chapter 5, treatment for encephalitis is largely "supportive," aimed at easing the symptoms and trying to help the patient's immune system help itself. With the exception of a small group of antiviral medications such as acyclovir, the best "treatment" for encephalitis is prevention. There are various ways to prevent encephalitis. For example, to prevent encephalitis from an arbovirus, the recommended strategy is to avoid mosquito bites by wearing insect repellant and protective clothing, staying indoors during peak mosquito hours, and having window screens at home to keep out mosquitoes. Another major prevention strategy is to eliminate the vector—namely mosquitoes. Aggressive aerial spraying of pesticides to kill mosquitoes has been undertaken in most regions seriously affected by West Nile virus and the encephalitis that often accompanies it.

Because many pathogens such as viruses are highly contagious, viral infections can affect whole communities, not just individual people. As a result, governmental agencies exist at the local, state, federal, and international levels that take responsibility for monitoring infectious diseases, administering vaccines (when available) to prevent them, advising the public on proper environmental and behavioral strategies to avoid infections, and conducting scientific research to develop new therapeutic and preventative measures.

PUBLIC HEALTH DEPARTMENTS IN THE
UNITED STATES: LOCAL, STATE, AND FEDERAL

Local health departments are the front line in monitoring, treating, and preventing infectious diseases such as viruses that cause encephalitis. New York City has one of the oldest and largest departments of health in the country—it was founded in 1866 and had organized predecessors dating back as far as 1655! In New York City, where the first American outbreak of West Nile virus took place, the Department of Health and Mental Hygiene maintains a list of infectious diseases that health-care providers must report. The department's Bureau of Communicable Diseases is responsible for responding to these reports. For example, during the mosquito breeding season (June–October), all cases of viral encephalitis must be reported immediately by phone or fax. The bureau investigates each case reported, communicates with physicians about various disease outbreaks, establishes standard practices for laboratory testing, dispenses information such as updates, and develops preventative measures such as pesticide spraying plans.

Each state has its own department of health, which typically helps coordinate the efforts of the various local departments around the state and sets priorities for the state as a whole. The state department of health provides information to consumers on health-care providers; immunization; long-term care; child, family, and senior health; and medical insurance.

At the federal level, the main agency for matters related to public health is the Centers for Disease Control and Prevention (CDC), which has its main headquarters in Atlanta, Georgia. Established in 1946 as part of the Department of Health and Human Services, the CDC's goal is to "promote health and quality of life by preventing and controlling disease, injury, and disability." The CDC works in collaboration with state and international governments. It has employees in 45 foreign

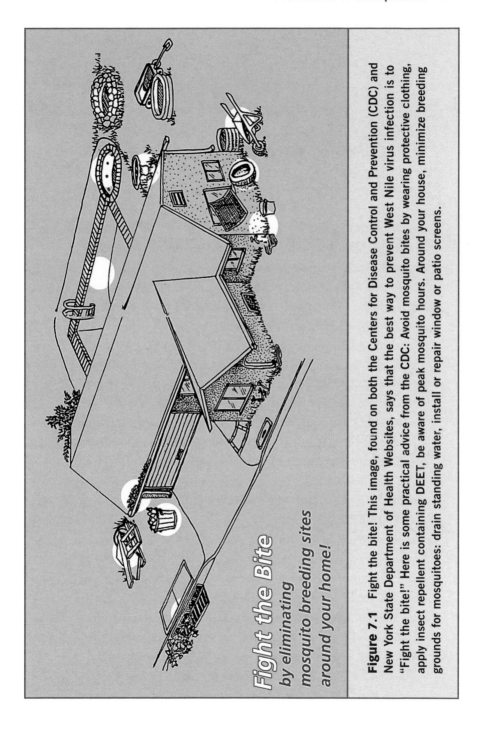

Figure 7.1 Fight the bite! This image, found on both the Centers for Disease Control and Prevention (CDC) and New York State Department of Health Websites, says that the best way to prevent West Nile virus infection is to "Fight the bite!" Here is some practical advice from the CDC: Avoid mosquito bites by wearing protective clothing, apply insect repellent containing DEET, be aware of peak mosquito hours. Around your house, minimize breeding grounds for mosquitoes: drain standing water, install or repair window or patio screens.

countries. The CDC coordinates the monitoring of diseases nationwide, including prevention effectiveness. The CDC maintains many offices or centers that are specifically dedicated to studying the viruses that can cause encephalitis, including HIV, measles, respiratory and enteric viruses, West Nile virus, and influenza. In addition, the CDC maintains the EMERGEncy ID NET. This is a collaborative network with the National Center for Infectious Diseases and is led by 11 university-affiliated, city hospital emergency departments that see close to 1 million patients among them each year. The network monitors the frequency of symptoms caused by infectious organisms such as the bacterium *Escherichia coli* (*E. coli*). It also specifically tracks encephalitis.

The CDC maintains a National Notifiable Diseases Surveillance System for state health departments to report cases of diseases "for which regular, frequent, and timely information regarding individual cases is considered necessary for the prevention and control of the disease." The list of diseases started in 1878 and included cholera, smallpox, plague, and yellow fever. It is reviewed and revised periodically. As of 2002, the list contained more than 50 infectious diseases, including viruses that can cause encephalitis, such as rabies, yellow fever, measles, mumps, HIV, and West Nile virus.

PUBLIC HEALTH DEPARTMENTS WORLDWIDE: WHAT IS THE WHO?

The World Health Organization, founded in 1948, is a branch of the United Nations (UN). It was designed to be the UN agency responsible for health-related services. The major objective of the WHO is to promote the highest level of health for all people. The definition of *health* used in the constitution of WHO is a "state of total physical, mental, and social well-being"—not just an absence of disease. An assembly of representatives from 192 countries governs the WHO, setting its priorities and budget. This international organization gathers data on infectious diseases such as encephalitis from around the world and works to monitor, treat, and prevent disease on a global level. The WHO's enormous database can generate maps of areas where there are outbreaks of infectious diseases and indicate such relevant information as the location of roads, schools, and health facilities. The WHO also keeps track of statistics regarding infectious diseases such as yellow fever and other viruses that cause encephalitis worldwide. In addition to monitoring diseases, the WHO also maintains a Global Outbreak Alert and Response Network (GOARN). This agency coordinates scientific, medical, and humanitarian groups to identify, confirm, and respond to outbreaks of infectious diseases.

VACCINATION AS A STRATEGY FOR PREVENTING ENCEPHALITIS

Here is a riddle for you: What does a cow have to do with acquiring immunity against a virus or other pathogen? Answer: The word *vaccine* comes from the Latin word for "cow," *vaca*. The first vaccine was developed using a virus called cowpox, which could infect cows as well as humans. (Scientists now call it *vaccinia* virus.) The cowpox virus was closely related to the smallpox (*variola*) virus, a highly contagious and deadly pathogen for which there is no cure. In the late 18th century, an English doctor named Edward Jenner realized that the women who worked on farms milking cows often got cowpox from the cows, but did not catch smallpox, even when the disease was rampant where they lived. Jenner hypothesized that the less severe cowpox infection somehow protected the women from smallpox infections. In an experiment that would not be permitted today due to ethical and human rights concerns, Jenner **inoculated** a healthy boy with cowpox. That is, he intentionally introduced the cowpox virus into the boy's body with the aim to provoke a mild disease response that would protect the body against both cowpox and smallpox (if his hypothesis was correct) later in life. A month and a half later, Jenner subjected the boy to infection with smallpox. Luckily for the boy, Jenner's hypothesis was correct, and the boy did not come down with a smallpox infection. In the 1950s, 50 million people worldwide contracted smallpox each year. In 1967, the WHO began a massive immunization campaign to try to eliminate the disease from the planet. Millions of children were vaccinated against smallpox, and the disease was successfully eradicated. The last natural case of smallpox occurred in 1977 in Somalia.

Vaccine Strategies

In order for a vaccine to be effective it must be safe, be protective in both the short and long term, and be practical to deliver. In other words, it has to provoke an adaptive immune response that leads to the establishment of antibodies and memory cells; must have few, if any, side effects; must be easy to make, ship, store, and use.

The principle of the smallpox vaccine introduced by Edward Jenner in the 1700s is still in use in some vaccines today—inoculation with a live but weakened (attenuated) virus in order to provoke an immune reaction. **Live attenuated viral vaccines** are as close to live, infectious viruses as can be prepared in the laboratory and given to people without causing serious disease. However, because live attenuated viruses are just that—alive—there is an inherent danger that the viruses may change (mutate) into a more infectious (virulent) form. Therefore, several other vaccine strategies have been developed—all of which are pertinent to overcoming infections that can cause encephalitis. For many viruses that can cause encephalitis, such as herpes simplex, HIV, and West Nile virus, research is under way using several of these strategies.

One vaccine strategy in use is to immunize a person with a virus that has been killed or inactivated using chemicals, heat, or irradiation (exposing something to radiation other

VACCINE AGAINST A CNS VIRUS: A SUCCESS STORY

In the 1950s, before the polio vaccine was developed, 50,000 new cases of polio were reported every year in the United States alone. Almost half of the victims became paralyzed. In 1955, Dr. Jonas Salk developed a vaccine against polio from inactivated polio virus that rapidly decreased the number of polio cases to 3,000 that same year. In 1962, Dr. Albert Sabin developed a vaccine from a live weakened virus that could be delivered orally. Because the poliovirus normally resides in the gastrointestinal system, introducing a vaccine to the gut proved to be extremely potent in producing immunity. Because it is made with a live virus, the Sabin vaccine causes about 1 out of every 2.4 million people immunized in the United States to contract polio and develop paralysis. Given that the risk for contracting polio is currently extremely low in the United States, the risk of the Sabin vaccine is now considered unnecessary, and the Salk vaccine is given instead. In 2001, the World Health Organization reported only 480 cases of polio worldwide and was well on its way to its goal of eradicating the disease altogether. However, progress has not been as quick as would be hoped. In 2003, the Nigerian government suspended some polio vaccine programs when local clergymen made the false claim that it was intended to sterilize girls and may contain HIV contaminants. An epidemic quickly broke out. Nigeria has since experienced more than 1,000 cases of polio. Due to civil war and unrest, some other African countries also suspended polio vaccination and case numbers quickly rose. With the reestablishment of an aggressive vaccination campaign, 80 million children were vaccinated in Africa in 2004, which should have a dramatic effect on stemming the emerging polio epidemic.

than that from visible light—for example, X rays). In this scenario, the immune system encounters most of the same ingredients as it would with a live virus. However, the immune response to a **killed virus** or **inactivated virus** is usually weaker. As a result, additional "booster" shots are often needed to get the immune system elevated to the correct level. This can be a drawback in communities where the health-care delivery system is not well developed, and it also increases the cost per dose of a vaccine—an important issue when millions of doses are being delivered.

Another strategy is to use just small pieces of the microbe, called antigens or **subunits**, of the microbe in question as the immunizing material. This process is very safe, because the person being immunized does not have an actual infectious organism in his or her body. However, the drawback is that microbes can mutate very rapidly, so the material used to immunize the person may become less useful over time. To address this issue, subunit vaccines often utilize a combination of several antigens from the same microbe, in the hope that giving the immune system more information about the microbe to use in creating memory cells is better. This is the kind of vaccine currently used to immunize people against the hepatitis B virus.

Sometimes, the pathogen in question secretes a substance that is particularly harmful, or toxic, to the host. In cases like this, scientists try to make the toxin in the laboratory, chemically inactivate it, and then use it instead of the actual microbe as the immunizing material. This is called a **toxoid vaccine**, and when it is used the host learns to fight the toxin without getting sick from it. Similarly, **conjugate vaccines** couple an antigen or toxoid with a sugar molecule. This is done to protect against some organisms (most often bacteria) that use a sugar coating to disguise themselves from the immune system. The host sees the toxin or antigen and also learns to recognize the sugar to which it is attached.

DNA vaccines are a recent and interesting development. In this strategy, the genome of a virus or other pathogen is the key to producing immunity. As you read in Chapter 2, many viral genomes have been decoded. Using this information, scientists can design pieces of viral DNA to be introduced to a person's immune system. The immune cells then respond to the viral DNA in the same way they would if they were actually infected by the whole virus. That is, cells immunized with a piece of viral DNA make some viral products, which they also then display on their surfaces. Just as with antigens from a real viral infection, the immune system learns to recognize these viral products. DNA vaccines are currently being tested for protection against HIV, herpes, and influenza viruses. Scientists are also working to develop DNA vaccines against West Nile virus.

Recombinant vector vaccines are a combination of the DNA vaccine and live virus vaccine strategy. Scientists take a nonpathogenic virus and change it to produce some of the antigens found in a harmful virus. When a person is immunized with this material, the immune system usually has a very robust response, similar to what occurs when a natural pathogen enters the body. Thus, the immune system learns to recognize pieces of the pathogenic virus without having to overcome a harmful virus infection. This strategy is being tested for HIV, rabies, and measles viruses.

Vaccines are often given in combination with chemical compounds called **adjuvants**, which help activate the immune response. Adjuvants work by keeping the vaccine material at the site of injection longer than it would normally stay and then helping the antigens travel to the lymph nodes, where adaptive immunity comes into play. In the United States, the only kind of adjuvant currently in use for people is called aluminum salt. Some pathogen-derived toxins, such as pertussis toxin, made by the bacteria that cause whooping cough, are adjuvants themselves and are given in combination with vaccinations against tetanus and diphtheria toxins.

We probably all have some unpleasant childhood memories of getting our vaccination shots in the pediatrician's office. The injection route of vaccine administration is not only sometimes painful but it is also costly. In addition to studying different kinds of vaccines, scientists are also trying to develop new and effective routes of vaccine administration that are less invasive and easier to deliver, store, and produce. In the future, many vaccines will probably be given in the form of a nasal spray, a skin patch, or something that may simply be eaten.

Production of Vaccines

Vaccines are regulated in the United States by the same federal agency that regulates all drugs sold to the public, the Food and Drug Administration (FDA). Before selling a vaccine, a pharmaceutical company must first test the vaccine in animals to show that it is safe and looks promising in protecting against the relevant infection (Table 7.1). Then the company can submit an application to the FDA describing the vaccine, its safety, and any data collected so far. If the company's application to investigate a new drug is approved, it can begin to test the safety of the vaccine on 20 human volunteers—this is called a phase I trial. In a phase II trial, 50 people can be treated with the vaccine to try to gather more safety data, test the vaccine's effectiveness, and arrive at a proper dose. In phase III clinical trials, thousands of people are treated with the vaccine and its effectiveness and safety must be clearly shown. If the vaccine is approved, the FDA continues to monitor its use in phase IV studies that pick up rare side effects or problems not seen in earlier studies. Throughout its use, a vaccine is routinely retested for its safety, purity, and effectiveness.

Table 7.1 Timeline for New Drug Development

CLINICAL RESEARCH AND DEVELOPMENT

	Years	Test Subjects	Purpose
Preclinical Testing, Research, and Development	1–3; average is 18 months	Laboratory and animal studies	Determine safety and biological activty
File IND* at FDA			
Phase I	Several months to 1 year	20 to 100 healthy volunteers	Determine safety
Phase II	Several months to 2 years	About 100 to 300 patient volunteers	Evaluate effectiveness; look for side effects
Phase III	1–4 years	Several hundred to several thousand patient volunteers	Confirm safety, effectiveness, and dosage
File NDA† at FDA			
FDA Review	Average 2.5 years	Review process and approval	
	12 Total		
Post-marketing Surveillance	Additional post-marketing testing by the FDA		

* IND = Investigational new drug application
† NDA = New drug application

The benefits of vaccination far outweigh the risks of getting any of the illnesses in question. Recently, some concerns have been raised about a connection between vaccination and the development of diseases such as autism and multiple sclerosis. Scientists and health authorities have studied the issue and determined that there is no tie between vaccines and these conditions.

8

Scientific Research and the Future of Encephalitis

SCIENTIFIC RESEARCH

Viruses can mutate over time, so the more knowledge we have of basic virology and of viral interactions with the immune system, the more likely we will be to develop effective vaccines against encephalitis-causing diseases and treatments for encephalitis. There are many institutions in the United States and around the world that conduct scientific and medical virology research including public and private universities, nonprofit institutes, commercial companies, and government-funded institutions. So who funds the science that helps us battle viral encephalitis?

The National Institutes of Health

The National Institutes of Health (NIH), founded in 1887, is headquartered in Bethesda, Maryland. It is the major agency for medical research in the United States. Like the CDC, the NIH is also part of the Department of Health and Human Services. Its goal is to pursue knowledge of living organisms and apply that knowledge to help promote health and reduce the incidence of illness. To do this, the NIH has 27 different institutes and centers, many of which fund the study of topics related to encephalitis. Of particular relevance to research on encephalitis are the NIH's National Institute of Allergy and Infectious Diseases (NIAID), the Office of AIDS Research (AOR), and the National Institute of Neurological Disorders and Stroke (NINDS).

RESEARCH FOUNDATIONS

In addition to the National Institutes of Health, there are many organizations and foundations that sponsor scientific research. One notable example is the Howard Hughes Medical Institute (HHMI), which was founded in 1953 by Howard R. Hughes, a founding father of the airplane industry. (A portrayal of Hughes's life can be seen in the 2004 movie *The Aviator*, starring Leonardo DiCaprio as Hughes.) The HHMI gives financial support to scientists who are preeminent in their fields. To date, the HHMI has provided more than $1 billion toward medical research.

Current Research Topics Related to Encephalitis

There are many scientific questions to be answered with regard to viruses and other pathogens that cause encephalitis. Learning the answers to these questions could lead to development of vaccines, antiviral medications, and better laboratory diagnostic tests for encephalitis. What kinds of immune system cells get into the brain during an infection of the central nervous system? How do they get into the brain during an infection? Which molecules are important for allowing viruses to cross the blood-brain barrier? How do latent viruses get reactivated? What are the best ways to vaccinate against viruses that cause encephalitis? What chemical compounds interfere specifically with viral replication and entry into cells but do not harm the host? These are just some of the questions related to encephalitis that remain to be answered. With ongoing research, perhaps scientists will someday find a way to stop encephalitis from claiming any more lives.

Appendix

VACCINE SAFETY

For reliable information about vaccine safety, the National Institutes of Health recommends contacting these organizations:

American Council on Science and Health
212-362-7044
www.acsh.org

Centers for Disease Control and Prevention
1-800-232-2552
www.cdc.gov

Immunization Safety Review Committee of the Institute of Medicine
202-334-1342
www.iom.edu/imsafety

Johns Hopkins University Institute of Vaccine Safety
www.vaccinesafey.edu

National Network for Immunization Information
1-877-341-6644
www.immunizationinfo.org

Vaccine Education Center at the Children's Hospital of Philadelphia
215-590-9990
www.vaccine.chop.edu

Glossary

Acute phase proteins—Proteins present in the blood during the earliest stages of infection or inflammation that help in the attempt to fight off the infection.

Adaptive immune system—The part of the immune system that develops throughout life and has an ability to change, expand, and remember specific immunological events.

Adjuvant—A chemical or compound that enhances the immune response to an antigen.

Amygdala—An almond-shaped region deep within the cerebral hemispheres of the brain that coordinates emotion, behavior and some kinds of learning and memory.

Antibody—A unique protein that binds to a specific substance (antigen) made by plasma cells in response to an infection or vaccination. These proteins can bind to pathogens or their antigens and neurtralize them directly, or they can flag them for destruction by other white blood cell types.

Antigen—A molecule that interacts specifically with antibodies or receptors on B or T cells.

Antigen presentation—The mechanism used by some cells to alert other cells of the immune system of the molecular nature of a specific pathogen or foreign substance. These "antigen presenting cells" display partial fragments of the pathogen or substance, called antigens, on their surface, which other cells can then detect.

Arbovirus—Arthropod borne virus; any virus that is spread by arthropods-usually blood-sucking insects such as ticks and mosquitoes.

Asymptomatic—Not showing symptoms.

Axons—A long and single nerve cell process that conducts impulses (usually from the cell body) to other nerve cells (neurons).

Bacteria (singular is **bacterium**)—Microorganisms that are usually single-celled and do not have a nucleus. There are thousands of different species of bacteria, most of which fall into three different shape categories: rod-like, round balls, and spiral. Some bacteria are harmful to humans and are therefore called pathogens, while other kinds peacefully co-exist with their human hosts.

Basal Ganglia—A region deep within the cerebral hemispheres of the brain that regulates movement of the body.

B cells—A type of lymphocyte which matures in the bone marrow and is the source of antibodies.

Bind—To attach to something such as when a virus or antigen attaches to a receptor on a cell surface.

Biopsy—The removal of a small piece of tissue for molecular and cellular analysis and examination.

Blood brain barrier—A barrier created by brain capillaries that prevents many substances from leaving the blood and crossing the capillary walls into the brain.

Brain stem—The part of the brain connecting the spinal cord and the cerebrum. This region includes the mesencephalon, pons, and medulla oblongata.

Capsid—The outer protein shell of a virus particle.

Capsomeres—The cluster of proteins that make up the basic coat of a viral genome.

Cell body—The nucleus-containing central part of a neuron exclusive of its axon and dendrite. The term may be used to describe the nucleus-containing part of other cell types as well.

Cell-mediated immunity—Relating to or being part of the immune response that is primarily mediated by antigen-specific T cells.

Cell membrane—The part of the cell that separates it from the outside environment. The membrane is flexible and made up mostly of lipids and proteins.

Central dogma-(of molecular biology)—The genetic information flow from DNA to RNA to protein.

Central nervous system (CNS)—The part of the body that in vertebrates consists of the brain and spinal cord. This organ is responsible for coordinating the entire activity of the animal.

Cerebellum—A brain structure that is attached to the brain stem and is important in controlling movement, including coordination of muscles and maintenance of balance.

Cerebral cortex—The layer directly below the cerebrum that functions to coordinate sensory and motor information.

Cerebral hemisphere—The two sides of the cerebrum, which is the largest region of the forebrain.

Glossary

Cerebrospinal Fluid (CSF)—A fluid that circulates throughout the CNS. It provides nutrition and also cushions the brain from impacts from the outside world. CSF is made in a region within the brain ventricles called the choroids plexus.

Chemokine—A kind of chemical signal released by macrophages or other immune cell types when encountering a pathogen or other pro-inflammatory stimuli. These molecules activate cells to migrate or change their behavior in response to a particular situation.

Choroid plexus—An area within each brain ventricle that makes cerebrospinal fluid.

Clone—(within the context of the immune system) The identical copies of a B or T cell that is generated in a response to a particular antigen that activated a specific B or T cell.

Complement—A group of proteins found in normal blood serum and plasma that helps to control inflammation and infection. It can be activated by antibodies and can also help lead to the productive neutralization of substances or pathogens by antibodies.

Conjugate vaccine—An immunization cocktail created by scientists that couples an antigen or toxin to a sugar molecule.

Co-receptor—A cell surface molecule that is needed in order for certain substances to transmit signals into the cell and may be used by some pathogens such as some types of viruses to gain entry into a cell.

Cytokine—A general term to describe a large variety of proteins secreted by activated cells that serves as local signaling molecules during inflammation, infection, or wound healing.

Cytotoxic—Of or relating to a substance that is poisonous (toxic) to cells.

Cytotoxic T lymphocyte—see **Killer T cell**.

Demyelination—The destruction of myelin, the insulating material surrounding the axons of many types of neurons. This demyelination is often due to an autoimmune disease and can have very unfavorable effects on the general nervous system function of a patient.

Dendrite—A relatively short, branched process of a nerve cell that receives information from other nerve cells.

Dendritic cells—White blood cells that develop in the bone marrow and then live in an "immature" state in the blood, tissues, skin, and mucosa throughout the body, where they serve as watchdogs of the immune system, constantly taking in material from the microenvironment around them, thus surveying the area.

Deoxyribonucleic acid (DNA)—A macromolecule in the shape of a double helix, found in the nucleus of cells and is thought to be the carrier of hereditary information.

Diencephalon—The posterior subdivision of the forebrain.

DNA vaccines—An immunization developed by scientists using a piece of DNA of a pathogen such as a virus to be encountered by the host's immune system.

Echovirus—see **Enterovirus**.

Encephalitis—An acute inflammation of the brain that can be caused by infectious agents such as a virus.

Encephalomyelitis—An acute inflammation of the brain and spinal cord.

Endocytosis—The ingestion of material from outside the cell by folding in of the cell membrane and swallowing it up along with the membrane.

Endothelial cells—Cells that line blood and lymphatic vessels.

Enterovirus—This group of viruses includes the poliovirus, Coxsackie viruses, and echoviruses, establish infection within the gastrointestinal (enteric) tract. Enteroviruses have genomes made of RNA, like many of the other viruses that can cause encephalitis, which enter the host cell, get copied and then translated into proteins needed for RNA synthesis.

Envelope (viral)—A layer of lipids and proteins that protects and surrounds a viral capsid and genome.

Epidemiology—The collective conditions and factors that influence the presence or absence of a disease or pathogen. This word also refers to the study of an epidemic, a disease that is prevalent at a particular time and place that is not usually present among a population.

Epithelia (singular is epithelium)—The membranous cellular tissues that line the cavities of the body and serve to enclose and protect the other parts of the body, to produce secretions and excretions.

Etiology—The underlying causes of a disease or abnormal condition.

Extracellular Fluid—Fluid that is outside of and in between cells.

Frontal lobe—A part of the brain involved in solving problems, planning, organization, working memory, emotions.

Glossary

Fusion—The merging or combination of distinct biological entities, like two membranes.

Genome—All of the genetic material of a particular organism.

Glia—Non-neuronal cells of the nervous system that function to support neurons.

Helper T cells—T cells that have a cell surface molecule called "CD4"; they help B cells make antibodies, activate killer T cells, and help mount many aspects of the adaptive immune response.

Hippocampus—An area of the cerebral cortex that plays a crucial role in learning and memory.

Host—A living organism that harbors or supports the existence of another organism, such as a parasite.

Hummoral immunity—The immune response that involves antibodies secreted by B cells and circulating in fluids within the body.

Immunological memory—Cells of the adaptive immune system that remain after the infection is resolved, that can quickly respond when the same organism is encountered again, making high titers of antibodies or lots of specific T cells.

Inactivated virus—A virus that has been treated with chemical, heat, or irradiation to render it unable to replicate on its own. Some vaccines include inactivated viruses in order to stimulate the immune system but avoid an infection.

Inflammation—A cellular response that is marked by capillary dilatation, leukocytic infiltration, redness, heat, and pain that serves as a mechanism initiating the elimination of noxious agents, pathogens, or the isolation of damaged tissue.

Innate immune system—The non-specific part of the immune system that exists at birth, usually remains unchanged throughout life, and is maintained by the skin and mucosa, (so-called "barriers" to infection), as well as by antimicrobial substances made by cells and by phagocytic cells which seek to destroy the offending pathogen or substance.

Inoculate—The introduction of a pathogen or substance that has been weakened or at a low dose in order to induce a mild immune response. This immune response will provide immunological memory via cells of the adaptive immune response, and will provide protection against the pathogen or substance during later encounters.

Interferons—A kind of cell-cell signaling molecule that provide some protection against viruses, made by cells exposed to a virus or sometimes to another kind of parasite or foreign organisms.

Killed virus—A virus that has been rendered unable to replicate or live within a host by treatment with chemicals, heat, or irradiation. Sometimes a vaccine can include a killed virus with the hopes of exposing the immune system to virus ingredients without the risk of a real infection.

Killer T cell—A T cell that has a surface molecule called "CD8" and can kill other cells including those infected by viruses.

Latent viral infection—A viral infection that is in a state of dormancy and is usually not detected by the immune system. Latent viruses can become re-activated by many factors such as stress, hormonal changes, and sunlight.

Leukocytes—A white blood cell.

Lipid—A molecule that does not dissolve in water. Lipids are the basis of all cell membranes.

Live attenuated viral vaccine—An immunization containing the a virus that is close to that found in nature but has been somewhat weakened by scientists in the laboratory.

Lymphocyte—A white blood cell that mediates the adaptive immune response such as T and B cells. These cells originate from stem cells and develop in lymphoid tissues such as bone marrow and thymus. These cells make up 20–30% of the white blood cells in normal human blood.

Lyse (noun form is **lysis**)—Disintegration or destruction of cells; lysis is the bursting of cells.

Macrophage—A cell of the innate immune system that develops from stem cells in the bone marrow and functions to protect the body against invasion by foreign substances or pathogens.

Major histocompatability complex (**MHC**)—A group of genes that encode highly variable proteins that sit on the surface of cells and bind pieces of foreign material to show them to T and B cells to induce an adaptive immune response. These proteins are involved in the molecular discrimination of "self" and "non-self" and are therefore key to healthy functioning of a person.

Meningitis—An inflammation of the protective membranes (called the meninges) surrounding the brain and spinal cord.

Glossary

Microbial—Having to do with microbes, which are life forms too small to be seen without the aid of a microscope.

Microglia—A kind of glia that serves as the resident macrophages of the nervous system.

Molecular mimicry—The process whereby a pathogen such as a virus makes the same or similar versions of molecules made by cells of the host they are infecting.

Motor systems—The systems that control voluntary skeletal muscle movements.

Mucosa—The mucus-coated lining of particular organs, such as the nose, mouth, lung, intestinal, and genital tracts.

Mutation—A change in the genetic information of an organism that may be inheritable and results in an altered gene or gene product.

Myelin—A soft white fatty material that surrounds the core of a nerve fiber and provides insulation.

Natural Killer cells (NK)—A kind of white blood cell that can specifically recognize a cell infected with a virus and release cytotoxic molecules to destroy it.

Neuroglia—see **Glia.**

Neuron (nerve cell)—A cell with specialized processes to send and receive information in the nervous system.

Neutrophil—A white blood cell that is specialized for phagocytosis and is typically a "first responder" cell type to a site of infection or inflammation.

Nucleocapsid—The nucleic acid and surrounding protein coat of a virus.

Nucleotide—Any of several compounds that consist of a ribose or deoxyribose sugar joined to a purine or pyrimidine base and to a phosphate group. These molecules are the basic structural units of nucleic acids like DNA and RNA.

Occipital lobe—Brain regions that control the organization of the visual information, such as how we see light and objects and how we recognize things.

Olfactory neuron—Nervous system cells that contribute to the sense of smell.

Parasite—A harmful organism that cannot live on its own but must live in another organism. Organisms that do this but do not harm their hosts are referred to as "symbiotic."

Parietal lobe—Region of the brain involved in interpreting sensory signals such as those that are associated with seeing, hearing, and touch.

Pathogen—A specific harmful infectious organism like a virus or bacteria that leads to the development of pathological changes in the host.

Phagocyotosis—The mechanism that a cell uses to ingest particulate matter from outside itself. (From the Greek word "*phagein*", meaning "to eat.")

Pleocytosis—The presence in the blood of an abnormally high number of white blood cells.

Poliovirus—An enterovirus that occurs in several strains of which one is the most frequent cause of human poliomyelitis, a disease characterized by fever, motor paralysis, and atrophy of skeletal muscles, often with permanent disability and deformity marked by inflammation of nerve cells in the spinal cord (encephalitis).

Pore—A small opening by which matter passes through a membrane.

Receptor—A molecule on the surface of a cell that interacts with a specific biological substance such as a chemical group, signaling molecule, or pathogen like a virus and can relay information to the inside of the cell.

Recombinant vector vaccine—A combination of a DNA vaccine and a live virus vaccine strategy.

Reservoir—An intermediate piece species in an arboviral transmission life cycle that can become infected and transmit the virus to another species.

Ribonucleic acid (RNA)—A single-stranded macromolecule that carries out DNA's instructions for protein synthesis.

Sensory system—The part of the body conveying nerve impulses from the sense organs to the nerve centers.

Sera (singular is **serum**)—The fluid part of the blood.

Spinal cord—The nervous tissue that extends from the brain lengthwise along the back in the vertebral canal, gives off the spinal nerves, carries impulses to and from the brain, and serves as a center for initiating and coordinating many reflex as well as other motor acts.

Stem cells—Undifferentiated cells that can give rise to other cell types.

Synapse—The place where two neurons connect and communicate with each other.

Glossary

T cells—A type of lymphocyte that matures in the thymus and directs cell-mediated immunity.

Temporal lobe—Area of the brain that is involved in processing sounds and their meanings. The temporal lobes are also involved in language, speech, and memory.

Toxoid vaccine—An immunization containing an inactivated toxin that was derived or created in the laboratory.

Trigeminal nerve—The nerve that provides most of the sensation to the face.

Tropism—In this biological context, the ability of a pathogen such as a virus, to selectively infect a particular type of cell. This propensity is usually based on a selective interaction with a receptor that is preferentially expressed on the infected cell type.

Vector—In this biological context, an intermediate host that does not become infected with an arbovirus but can spread the virus to another species.

Viremia—The concentration of virus particles in the blood. A higher viremia makes it easier for the infection to spread throughout the body.

Virion—A new virus particle produced as the virus replicates within a host cell.

Virus—A submicroscopic infectious organism that can range from the simple to the complex, that typically contains a protein coat surrounding an RNA or DNA core of genetic material but no semipermeable membrane. These organisms are capable of growth and muliplication only within other living cells and are therefore referred to as obligate intracellular parasites. Infection by some of these organisms can lead to many human diseases.

White blood cells—A mass of protoplasm that is colorless, lacks hemoglobin, contains a nucleus, and includes the lymphocytes, monocytes, neutrophils, eosinophils, and basophils.

Zoonotic—Capable of being spread from animal to humans under normal conditions.

Bibliography

BOOKS AND ARTICLES

Alberts, Bruce, Alexander Johnson, Julian Lewis, Martin Raff, Keith Roberts, and Peter Walter. *The Molecular Biology of the Cell.* New York: Garland Press, 2002.

Cann, Alan J. *Principles of Molecular Virology.* London, UK: Academic Press, 2001.

CDC Epidemic/Epizootic West Nile Virus in the United States; Guidelines for Surveillance, Prevention, and Control. U.S. Department of Health and Human Services, National Centers for Disease Control, National Center for Infectious Diseases, Division of Vector-Borne Infectious Diseases.

Cooper, Geoffrey M., and Robert E. Hausman. *The Cell: A Molecular Approach.* Sunderland, MA: Sinauer Associates, Inc., 2003.

Diamond, M. S., and R. S. Klein. "West Nile Virus: Crossing the Blood-Brain Barrier." *Nature Medicine* 10 (2004): 1294–1295.

Diamond, M. S., B. Shrestha, E. Mehlhop, E. Sitati, and M. Engle. "Innate and Adaptive Immune Responses Determine Protection against Disseminated Infection by West Nile Encephalitis Virus." *Viral Immunology* 16 (2003): 259–278.

Griffin, Diane E. "Immune Responses to RNA-Virus Infections of the CNS." *Nature Review Immunology* 3 (2003): 493–502.

Janeway, C., P. Travers, M. Walport, and M. Shlomchik. *The Immune System in Health and Disease.* New York: Garland Press, 2001.

Kandel, Eric R., James H. Schwartz, and Thomas M. Jessell. *Principles of Neural Science.* New York: McGraw-Hill/Appleton & Lange, 2000.

Kennedy, P.G.E. "Viral Encephalitis: Causes, Differential Diagnosis, and Management." *Journal of Neurology, Neurosurgery, and Psychiatry* 75 (2004): 10–15.

Koshiniemi, M., T. Rantahailo, H. Piiparinen, C. H. von Bonsdorff, M. Farkkila, A. Jarvinen, et al. "Infections of the Central Nervous System of Suspected Viral Origin: A Collaborative Study from Finland." *Journal of Neurovirology* 7(5) (2000): 400–408.

Lander, E. S., L. M. Linton, B. Birren, C. Nusbaum, M. C. Zody, J. Baldwin, K. Devon, et al. "Initial Sequencing and Analysis of the Human Genome." *Nature* 409 (2001): 860–921.

Bibliography

Nash, D., F. Mostashari, A. Fine, J. Miller, D. O'Leary, K. Murray, A. Huang, et al. "The Outbreak of West Nile Virus Infection in the New York City Area in 1999." *New England Journal of Medicine* 344 (2001): 1807–1814.

NIAID Science Education Brochure: Understanding Vaccines New York City Bureau of Communicable Diseases Polio Vaccine Fact Sheet.

Purves, Dale, George J. Augustine, David Fitzpatrick, Lawrence C. Katz, Anthony-Samuel Lamantia, James O. McNamara, and S. Mark Williams. *Neuroscience.* Sunderland, MA: Sinauer Associates, 2001.

Sejvar, James J., Maryam B. Haddad, Bruce C. Tierney, Grant L. Campbell, Anthony A. Marfin, Jay A. Van Gerpen, Aaron Fleischauer, et al. "Neurologic Manifestations and Outcome of West Nile Virus Infection." *Journal of the American Medical Association* 290 (2003): 511–515.

Solomon, T. "Current Concepts: Flavivirus Encephalitis." *New England Journal of Medicine* 351 (2004): 370–378.

Strauss, Ellen G., and James Strauss. *Viruses and Human Disease.* New York: Garland Press, 2001.

Tracey, K. J. "The Inflammatory Reflex." *Nature* 420 (2002): 853–859.

Tyler, K. L. "West Nile Virus Encephalitis in America." *New England Journal of Medicine* 344 (2001): 1858–1859.

Venter, J. Craig, Karin Remington, John F. Heidelberg, Aaron L. Halpern, Doug Rusch, Jonathan A. Eisen, et al. "Genome Shotgun Sequencing of the Sargasso Sea." *Science* 304 (2004): 66–74.

Venter, J. Craig, Mark D. Adams, Eugene W. Myers, Peter W. Li, Richard J. Mural, Granger Sutton, Hamilton O. Smith, et al. "The Sequence of the Human Genome." *Science* 291 (2001): 1304–1351.

Villareal, Luis P. "Are Viruses Alive?" *Scientific American* (December 2004): 100–105.

Wang, Tian, Eileen Scully, Zhinan Yin, Jung H. Kim, Sha Wang, Mark M. Mamula, John F. Anderson, Joe Craft, and Erol Fikrig. "IFN-Gamma-Producing Gamma Delta Cells Help Control Murine West Nile Virus Infection." *Journal of Immunology* 171 (2003): 2524–2531.

Wang, Tian, and Erol Fikrig. "Immunity to West Nile Virus." *Current Opinion in Immunology* 16 (2004): 519–523.

Wang, Tian, T. Town, L. Alexopoulou, J. F. Anderson, E. Fikrig, and R. A. Flavell. "Toll-Like Receptor 3 Mediates West Nile Virus Entry Into the brain Causing Lethal Encephalitis." *Nature Medicine* 10 (2004): 1366–1373.

Further Reading

BOOKS:

Carper, J. *Your Miracle Brain.* New York: HarperCollins Publishers, 2000.

Emmeluth, D. *Influenza.* Philadelphia: Chelsea House Publishers, 2003.

Ferreiro, C. *Mad Cow Disease (Bovine Spongiform Encephalopathy).* Chelsea House Publishers, 2005.

Kolb, B., and I.Q. Whislaw. *An Introduction to Brain and Behavior.* New York: Worth Publishers, 2001.

Levine, Arnold J. *Viruses.* Scientific American Library No. 37

Morgan, J., and O. Bloom. *Cells of the Nervous System.* Philadelphia: Chelsea House Publishers, 2005.

The Dana Foundation (www.dana.org) recommends:

Fleishman, J. *Phineas Gage: A Gruesome but True Story about Brain Science.* Boston: Houghton Mifflin, 2002.

Hayhurst, C. *The Brain and the Spinal Cord: Learning How We Think, Feel and Move.* New York: Rosen Publishing Group, 2002.

Landau, E. *Head and Brain Injuries.* Berkley Heights: Enslow Publishers, 2002.

Websites

Centers for Disease Control and Prevention
http://www.cdc.gov/

Current Health News
http://www.nlm.nih.gov/medlineplus/

Deadly Viruses
http://library.thinkquest.org/23054/basics/page7.html

Medical Terms
http://www.medterms.com/

National Institutes for Health
http://www.nih.gov/

New York City Department of Public Health
http://www.nyc.gov/html/doh/home.html

Viral Encephalitis
http://www.umm.edu/

Viruses
http://www.microbe.org/microbes/virus1.asp

Index

Index

Picture Credits

12: Courtesy CDC, *MMWR*, Vol 53, No 45; 1071 (11/19/2004)
19: © Dr. Gopal Murti/Visuals Unlimited
24: © Peter Lamb
26: © Peter Lamb
28: © Dr. Gopal Murti/Visuals Unlimited
34: © Peter Lamb
42: © Peter Lamb
43: © Peter Lamb
46: © Peter Lamb
52: © Peter Lamb
55: © Dr. John D. Cunningham/ Visuals Unlimited

56: © Peter Lamb
60: © Peter Lamb
63: © Peter Lamb
71: © Peter Lamb
72: © Mediscan/Visuals Unlimited
74: © Peter Lamb
83: © CORBIS
85: (middle) © Peter Lamb
85: (bottom)
    © Dr. Ken Greer/Visuals Unlimited
87: © Peter Lamb
91: Courtesy CDC

Cover: © Dr. F.A. Murphy/Visuals Unlimited

About the Authors

Ona Bloom is postdoctoral fellow at the Yale University School of Medicine. She has been interested at the interface between the nervous and immune systems since her senior year at Barnard College. She graduated with a B.A. degree in History from Barnard College in 1992 and began working as a research assistant under the supervision of Dr. Kevin J. Tracey, where she participated in his studies on the interactions between the immune and nervous systems. In 2001, Dr. Bloom earned her Ph.D from The Rockefeller University in New York City, under the supervision of Nobel Laureate Paul Greengard. Her doctoral work concentrated on the molecular anatomy of neuronal synapses.

Dr. Bloom is currently continuing her training at the Yale University School of Medicine under the supervision of Professor Ira Mellman in the departments of Cell Biology and Immunology. Dr. Bloom's fellowship has been funded by the National Institutes of Health and by the Cancer Research Institute. Currently, her scientific work focuses on the role of neuronal proteins at the immunological synapse, which is the place where antigen presenting cells communicate with lymphocytes. In the future, Dr. Bloom plans to continue working at the interface of the nervous and immune systems. When not at work, Dr. Bloom enjoys cooking, theater, music, and travel.

Jennifer Morgan is originally from Rutherfordton, North Carolina. She graduated in 1991 with highest honors from RS Central High School. From there, Jennifer went to the University of North Carolina at Chapel Hill. She began studying neurobiology during her sophomore year under the guidance of Dr. Ann Stuart. In 1995, she graduated with a Bachelor of Science degree with Honors in Biology. After taking a year off to continue her research, Jennifer began her graduate training at Duke University under the guidance of Dr. George Augustine. She earned a Ph.D. in Neurobiology in 2001. Dr. Morgan continues her training as a postdoctoral fellow in the laboratory of Dr. Pietro De Camilli at Yale University where she currently studies synaptic vesicle recycling. Her research has been supported by a Brown-Coxe Postdoctoral Fellowship (Yale), a Grass Fellowship in Neurosciences (Grass Foundation/MBL), and an individual postdoctoral National Research Service Award (NIH/NIMH). Throughout her career as a scientist, Jennifer has spent many summers doing research and teaching at the Marine Biological Laboratory in Woods Hole, MA. Last year, she was elected a member of the MBL Corporation. When she is not working, Jennifer enjoys singing and playing bass guitar in her band called 'The Secret Ink', traveling, and teaching her two cats to do tricks.

About the Founding Editor

The late I. Edward Alcamo was a Distinguished Teaching Professor of Microbiology at the State University of New York at Farmingdale. Alcamo studied biology at Iona College in New York and earned his M.S. and Ph.D. degrees in microbiology at St. John's University, also in New York. He had taught at Farmingdale for over 30 years. In 2000, Alcamo won the Carski Award for Distinguished Teaching in Microbiology, the highest honor for microbiology teachers in the United States. He was a member of the American Society for Microbiology, the National Association of Biology Teachers, and the American Medical Writers Association. Alcamo authored numerous books on the subjects of microbiology, AIDS, and DNA technology as well as the award-winning textbook *Fundamentals of Microbiology*, now in its sixth edition.